Atlas of Reproductive Surgery and Assisted Reproductive Technology Procedures

For Jim and Barb Marlay,
who truly believed anything is possible!

Atlas of Reproductive Surgery and Assisted Reproductive Technology Procedures

David S. McLaughlin MD

Reproductive Surgery and Medicine, P.C.

Indianapolis,

Indiana

USA

MARTIN DUNITZ

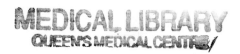
© **Martin Dunitz Ltd 2000**

First published in the United Kingdom in 2000
by Martin Dunitz Ltd, The Livery House,
7–9 Pratt Street, London NW1 0AE

A CIP record for this book is available from the British Library.

ISBN 1–85317–710–5

Distributed in the United States by:
Blackwell Science Inc.
Commerce Place, 350 Main Street
Malden, MA 02148, USA
Tel: 1-800-215-1000

Distributed in Canada by:
Login Brothers Book Company
324 Salteaux Crescent
Winnipeg, Manitoba, R3J 3T2
Canada
Tel: 204-224-4068

Distributed in Brazil by:
Ernesto Reichmann Distribuidora de Livros, Ltda
Rua Coronel Marques 335
03440-000 São Paulo–SP
Brazil

Composition by Scribe Design, Gillingham, Kent, UK
Printed and bound in Hong Kong by Imago.

Contents

Preface

This atlas is published for those healthcare providers who wish to offer their patients practical clinical state-of-the-art options to enhance or preserve their reproductive potential. The reproductive therapy chosen may be pursued as an immediate treatment for an infertile condition, as an option for a woman who wishes to consider pregnancy at a later date, or as an alternative for the patient who wishes to avoid hysterectomy. Once childbearing is complete, endometrial ablation for menorrhagia may be selected or definitive surgery may be accomplished by laparoscopic assisted vaginal hysterectomy (LAVH) with a shortened recovery time.

It is imperative that, as healthcare providers, we listen intently to each patient's concerns regarding her reproductive health prior to selecting the appropriate treatment option for her gynecological condition.

Acknowledgments

I am forever indebted to my family, Barb, Jeff, Scott, Molly, and Mark, who have continued to encourage me and support my efforts to formalize the experience I have gained through 25 years of developing expertise in reproductive surgery and assisted reproductive technology. I appreciate the opportunity, assistance, and expertise provided by my editors at Martin Dunitz Ltd, Robert Peden, Alan Burgess, and Mike Meakin. I wish to extend my sincere appreciation to those men and women who have enabled me to complete this atlas in a timely fashion: Barb Marlay, for her medical photographic expertise; Sharon Farrier, for her excellent manuscript preparation; Tim Campbell, for graphic illustrations; Joe Williams, Olympus Corporation, for technical photodocumentation assistance; Drs. Jim Daniell, Milton Goldrath, and Jack Lomano for clinical slides; Drs. Jerome Conia, Mitchell Schiewe, Beth Critser, Jeff Boldt, and Pat Schnaar for IVF laboratory assistance; and Bard, Ethicon, Genzyme, Gynecare Products, W.L. Gore, Laserscope, Laser Peripherals, Marlowe Surgical Technologies, Origin, Sharplan, Surgical Laser Technologies, Storz, Surgilase, Surgimedics, and U.S. Surgical for product slides. I do thank other scientists and physicians who have encouraged my interests in these fields: Alan Trounson, Gary Hodgen, Joe Feste, Dan Martin, Mickey Baggish, Bud Keye, and Michael Diamond. I also appreciate the opportunity to be selected to provide a one-year Fellowship in Reproductive Surgery, approved by the Society of Reproductive Surgeons through the American Society for Reproductive Medicine.

Introduction

History of gynecological endoscopy

Since medical history was first recorded until the present time, great strides in the advancement of techniques to help alleviate human pain and suffering have evolved. It seems as though a new idea was introduced by an innovative medical scholar, skepticism delayed acceptance into the medical mainstream, then technical advances were made in medical instrumentation, which subsequently led to widespread new applications by other investigators. Finally, scientific acceptance into the medical community evolved. Many pioneers pursued the refinement of their particular techniques in hysteroscopy (Table I.1), laparoscopy (Table I.2), and laser surgery (Table I.3). Ever since Pantaleoni visualized the endometrial cavity in a 60-year-old patient with post-menopausal bleeding in 1864, controversy ensued regarding gynecological endoscopy. This pioneer was censored by the Italian medical establishment for being 'too curious' when he initiated the first recorded diagnostic hysteroscopy. Many medical pioneers have had to overcome adversity to realize final acceptance by their medical peers. This atlas is dedicated to the spirit of those men and women who have enabled us to deliver gynecological care at the present state of the art, as well as to the new medical pioneers who will continue to hone the cutting edge with improved gynecological technology in the future.

Table I.1 **Hysteroscopy**

1869	Pantaleoni	First recorded diagnostic hysteroscopy
1925	Stern	Tungsten loop in a sheath carriage
1957	Norment	Therapeutic use of resectoscope for hysteroscopic myomectomy
1972	Neuwirth	Pioneered use to remove intra-uterine lesions and endometrial ablation
1981	Goldrath	Nd:YAG laser endometrial ablation
1983	DeCherney	Resectoscope management of uterine lesions and bleeding
1986	DeCherney	Transcervical metroplasty
1990	Townsend	Rollerball ablation

Table I.2 **Laparoscopy**

1910	Jacobeus	Cystoscope used to view intra-abdominal ascites
1911	Bernheim	Proctoscope with headlight
1920	Orndoff	Thoracoscope with oxygen pneumoperitoneum and local anesthesia for laparoscopy
1924	Steiner	Cystoscope, atmospheric air, with local anesthesia
1929	Kalk	Applied laparoscopy to internal medicine
1934	Ruddock	Recommended as a surgical procedure, developed biopsy forceps, accepted by gynecologists
1937	Hope	Used for ectopic pregnancy
1947	Fourestier	Cold-light illumination
1954	Palmer	No complications in 250 patients
1965	Frangenheim	Used general anesthesia
1967	Steptoe	First British publication
1968	Cohen	First American publication
1970	Wheeless	Popularized use for sterilization
1974	Semm	Popularized operative laparoscopy

Table I.3 **Lasers**		
1958	Schalow, Townes	Optical maser described
1960	Maimon	Ruby laser
1964	Patel	CO_2 laser
1973	Kaplan	CO_2 laser treatment of the cervix
1974	Bellina	Gynecological applications of CO_2 laser
1979	Bruhat	CO_2 laser laparoscopy in Europe
1981	Goldrath	Nd:YAG laser hysteroscopic endometrial ablation
1981	Baggish, Chong	Intra-abdominal aplication of CO_2 laser
1982	McLaughlin	Microlaser myomectomy with CO_2 laser
1982	Daniell	CO_2 laser laparoscopy in America
1983	Bellina	Microlaser tubal surgery with CO_2 laser
1983	Keye	Argon laser laparoscopy
1983	McLaughlin	Intra-abdominal surgical instruments
1985	Lomano	Nd:YAG laser laparoscopy
1986	Daniell	KTP laser laparoscopy

Conventional infertility evaluation and treatment

Nearly 8.4% of women during the reproductive years have difficulty conceiving. According to a survey by the National Center for Health Statistics, this included nearly 5 million women in 1988. Half had primary infertility; the other half had delivered at least one child. Nearly one-fourth of American women are affected, with about half of the infertile women currently seeking treatment. Women with primary infertility were twice as likely to seek treatment as those with secondary infertility. Half of the couples eventually conceive with their prognosis affected by duration of infertility, age of the woman, and etiology of the infertility. Although assisted reproductive technology (ART) has increased the pregnancy rate, treatment independent pregnancies occur at a rate of approximately 3% per month for those patients with idiopathic infertility.

In the US, multiple causes are documented: ovulation defects (16%), tubal factors (12%), male factors (18%), endometriosis (25%), and unexplained (17%). About 75% of the known causes may be detected by an initial evaluation consisting of a history, physical, semen analysis, hysterosalpin-

gogram (HSG), basal body temperature (BBT) chart, and laparoscopy. Additional testing may include *Chlamydia trachomatis*, *Ureaplasma urealyticum*, *Mycoplasma hominis*, strict morphologic criteria for spermatozoa with ovarian reserve testing (Day 3 FSH:Estradiol), hysteroscopy, and laparoscopy.

Empiric treatment with ovulation induction and possibly intra-uterine insemination remains unproved but it is a logical approach to help the infertile couple retain autonomy while recognizing their financial and emotional needs. If this course is selected, it is important to consider the woman's age and limit the course of treatment to three to four cycles. The chance for success diminishes by the patient's age (<30, 19%; 31–35, 13%; 36–40, 7%; and >41, 5%) and the duration of treatment (85% of pregnancies occurred within four treatment cycles). The American Society for Reproductive Medicine has issued a warning against prescribing clomiphene citrate for more than six cycles due to a possible increased risk of ovarian malignancy. A Canadian study reported that most patients were willing to tolerate a moderate increase in their lifetime risk for ovarian cancer due to fertility treatment, but most based their decision on a limited knowledge of the facts. A Danish study noted that nulliparity implies a 1.5 to 2-fold increased risk for ovarian cancer. Infertility without medical treatment increased this risk factor. Treatment with fertility drugs did not increase the ovarian cancer risk for women whether they conceived or not. Thus, for those women who are unsuccessful with clomiphene treatment, gonadotropin therapy may be an option, possibly combined with a gonadotropin agonist. This therapy requires more intensive monitoring (vaginal ultrasounds, serum estradiols, luteinizing hormone (LH), and progesterone) in order to achieve the appropriate dose and response. Follicle-stimulating hormone (FSH) therapy has an increased risk of multiple births (25%) and an increased chance of ovarian hyperstimulation syndrome (OHSS).

Endometriosis reduces the chance for conception to approximately 4% per month probably due to a factor present in the peritoneal fluid that impairs gamete function. Diagnostic laparoscopy remains the 'gold standard' used to diagnose this ubiquitous disease. The accuracy of laparoscopic diagnosis depends on the ability of the surgeon to recognize the disease. The peritoneal implants may be bluish-gray 'powder burns;' the darkened color is attributed to encapsulated menstrual blood. Endometrial implants may also appear as clear vesicles, white plaques, and reddish petechiae or flame-like areas. They range from several millimeters to 2 cm in diameter and may be superficial or deeply invasive. Chronic inflammation from the lesions may result in a fibrous reaction, causing local scarring and adhesion formation. Peritoneal pockets, Allen–Masters Syndrome, are commonly associated with endometrial implants. Microscopic lesions may also be present in the visually normal peritoneal lining, obscuring them from the gynecological surgeon.

Surgical vaporization of the endometrial implants increases the chance of conception and avoids drug side effects. Clinical studies indicate a significant loss in bone mineral density (up to 14%) after depot leuprolide therapy, recovering to a deficit of 4.2% at six months and 3.3% twelve months after therapy completion. Similar, but less severe, findings were confirmed in a study using nafarelin. Endometriosis-associated pain may be successfully treated with medical and/or surgical therapy, although neither therapy is efficacious in all patients. New research indicates that uterine receptivity to the embryo may be enhanced by treating with a gonadotropin agonist for three months post-operatively. The use of endometriosis-associated infertility treatment by medical therapy alone is not supported by the literature. Surgical treatment of this disease results in a cumulative pregnancy rate of approximately 52% with a recurrence rate of 28% within 18 months and 40% after nine years. ART offers hope for those patients who have not conceived with conventional therapy and may be considered earlier for those women with advanced age or endometrial stage.

The efficacy of conservative surgery for endometriosis-related pain is unclear. In several uncontrolled trials, the pain improvement rate was 70–100% immediately, decreasing to 82% at one year and 66% at five years. Until a greater understanding of this enigmatic disease is attained, selection of treatment will continue to be based not on one standard algorithm, but on individualized clinical judgment.

Tubal surgery pregnancy success for advanced disease has not greatly improved with evolving technology. ART may be justifiably considered an initial therapy, depending on the success rates of the tubal surgeon and the in vitro fertilization (IVF) program.

Assisted reproductive technology

Human IVF was first predicted in an unsigned editorial, presumably authored by Rock, published in 1937 in the New England Journal of Medicine. Seven years later, Rock and Menken reported the first successful IVF with human eggs. Shettles, an early pioneer in the field, was the first to realize the potential this therapy could have in treating infertile couples with damaged tubes. For these reasons, Glenister and Hamilton, professors of anatomy at the University of London, published a letter in The Times that the IVF birth of Louise Brown could not be 'acclaimed as new, nor as a British achievement.' The American researchers concentrated their work on fertilization and did not perform embryo transfer. The reasons given were the difficulty in obtaining oocytes (prior to laparoscopy) and the possible jeopardy in which it may place their institution in obtaining continued grants from the National Institutes of Health.

In vitro fertilization with embryo transfer (IVF-ET) was first successfully accomplished in rabbits in 1958 and then in humans in 1978. Patrick Steptoe, a British gynecologist in Oldham, Great Britain, pioneered a laparoscopic technique under the tutelage of Palmer, in France, and Frangenheim, in Germany, in the late 1950s. Edwards, knowledgeable in embryology, genetics, and immunology, read Steptoe's 1967 article in The Lancet, entitled 'Laparoscopy and Ovulation.' Six months later, Edwards was impressed by Steptoe's knowledge and how professionally he handled criticism at the Royal Society of Medicine's debate on the merits of laparoscopy. (Most of Edwards' gynecological friends had forewarned him that laparoscopy was an unacceptable procedure.) The two began their collaboration and soon after published their early work on 56 oocytes. The response was overwhelmingly critical in both the lay and scientific press. The BBC produced a television program about IVF which opened with a picture of the atomic bomb explosion at Hiroshima. The Archbishop of Liverpool denounced Steptoe's and Edwards' efforts as 'morally wrong.'

In 1971, they were denied long-term support for their research by the Medical Research Council. Subsequently, private sources, mostly from the United States, were tapped to initiate the first IVF laboratory at Kershaw's Hospital, about two miles north of Oldham. Through most of that decade not one patient conceived, resulting in years of frustration, disappointment, and scientific criticism. In particular, James Watson, who had recently been awarded the Nobel prize, condemned them on the grounds that they 'would produce monsters and make other mistakes.'

When Lesley and John Brown's daughter, Louise, was born in July, 1978, by Cesarean section (performed during the night under police guard), the world reacted as if she were a creature of science fiction. Now, 20 years later, she has emerged as a happy, healthy woman. Later that year, Steptoe and Edwards presented details of their work to the Royal College of Obstetricians and Gynaecologists in

London. They received a standing ovation, which had never occurred before. When Steptoe presented his data to the American Fertility Society in San Francisco later that year, the ovation at the conclusion of his lecture moved him to tears. After Louise Brown's birth, Steptoe and Edwards proclaimed their duty to get a thousand others like her, so she wouldn't be alone. Four years later, they had met their goal at their private clinic, Bourne Hall.

America's first IVF birth was Elizabeth Carr on December 28, 1981, a product of Georgeanna and Howard Jones' research, three years after initiating their IVF clinic at the Eastern Virginia Medical School. In 1985, 257 IVF births occurred in the United States; a decade later, there were 11,342 from 320 IVF clinics in the US. At present nearly 500,000 children around the world owe their lives to the technique of IVF-ET.

Currently, ART is therapeutic for almost all causes of infertility, especially if one includes donor eggs for those women with oocyte depletion, intracyto-plasmic sperm injection (ICSI) for severe male factor, and gestational surrogacy for women with an absent or severely malformed uterus.

The monthly chance of conception is greater with ART than any other treatment of infertility. Successive attempts may lead to pregnancy rates approaching 80%, although nearly two-thirds of the couples undertake an ART procedure only once. Currently, over 300 clinics in the US offer an ART procedure with the national published delivery rate in 1996 (Society of Assisted Reproductive Technology data) listed as 25.9%/retrieval for IVF and 28.7%/retrieval for gamete intrafallopian transfer (GIFT) (48,354 total attempts). More research is ongoing in order to positively influence the success rates while limiting the chance of multiple births, such as Day 5 blastocyst transfer. Due to the possible link of ovulation induction agents with epithelial ovarian tumors, patients should be appropriately evaluated, informed about possible long-term risks, and an efficient treatment plan initiated, then followed to obtain maximum benefit.

BIBLIOGRAPHY

Agarwal SK, Buyalos RP: Clomiphene citrate with intrauterine insemination: is it effective therapy in women above the age of 35 years? *Fertil Steril* **65**:759–63, 1996.

Anonymous. Miracle Babies. *People* **50**:62–9, 1998.

Dawood M, Ramos J, Khan-Dawood F: Depot leuprolide acetate versus danazol for treatment of pelvic endometriosis: changes in vertebral bone mass and serum estradiol and calcitonin. *Fertil Steril* **63**:1177–83, 1995.

Falcone T, Goldberg J, Miller K: Endometriosis: medical and surgical intervention. *Curr Opin Obstet Gynecol* **8**:178–83, 1996.

Jones HW, Jr., Toner JP: The infertile couple. *N Engl J Med* **329**:1710–15, 1993.

Lindemann HJ: 100 Years of Hysteroscopy: 1869 to 1969. In Siegler AM, Lindemann HG (eds): *Hysteroscopy Principles and Practice*. Philadelphia, J.B. Lippincott, p 11, 1984.

Litynski G, Steptoe PC: Laparoscopy, sterilization, the test-tube baby, and mass media. *J Soc Laparosc Surg* **2**:99–101, 1998.

Lu P, Ory S: Endometriosis: Current management. *Mayo Clin Proc* **70**:453–63, 1995.

Morales AJ, Murphy AA: Operative laparoscopy in gynecology. In: *Current Problems in Obstetrics, Gynecology and Fertility*. St. Louis, Mosby Year Book, Vol. 15, p 73, 1992.

Mosgaard B, Lidegaard O, Kjaer S, et al: Infertility, fertility drugs and invasive ovarian cancer: a case-control study. *Fertil Steril* **67**:1005–12, 1997.

Olive D, Schwartz L: Medical progress: endometriosis. *N Engl J Med* **328**:1759–69, 1993.

Orwoll E, Yuzpe A, Burry K, et al: Nafarelin therapy in endometriosis: long-term effects on bone mineral density. *Am J Obstet Gynecol* **171**:1221–5, 1994.

Rock J: Conception in a watch glass. *N Engl J Med* **217**:678, 1937.

Rosen B, Irvine J, Ritvo P, et al: The feasibility of assessing women's perceptions of the risks and benefits of fertility drug therapy in relation to ovarian cancer risk. *Fertil Steril* **68**: 90–4, 1998.

Shoham Z, Howles CM, Jacobs HS: Female Infertility Therapy. London, Martin Dunitz Ltd, 1999.

Shushan A, Paltiel O, Iscovich J: Human menopausal gonadotropin and the risk of epithelial ovarian cancer. *Fertil Steril* **65**:13–18, 1996.

Spiritas R, Kaufman S, Alexander N: Fertility drugs and ovarian cancer: Red alert or red herring? *Fertil Steril* **59**:291–3, 1993.

Torres JE: History of the laser. In McLaughlin DS (ed): *Lasers in Gynecology*. Philadelphia, J.B. Lippincott, p 3–6, 1991.

Venn A, Watson L, Lumley J, et al: Breast and ovarian cancer incidence after infertility and in vitro fertilisation. *Lancet* **346**:995–1000, 1995.

1 Getting started – the basics

Acquiring knowledge and skills

Acquiring new surgical skills as the technology revolution continues in gynecology can be a frustrating experience. Formal educational goals are attained during residency through learning didactic information while gradually acquiring technical expertise during supervised surgical experiences. Once in practice, the gynecologist needs to continue this method of learning, by assimilating published new techniques and attending didactic lectures as well as experiencing surgical hands-on laboratory training in post-graduate courses. Confidence in performing new techniques should be built as surgical responsibility is gradually increased during a preceptorship. Accrediting the gynecologist in the newly acquired surgical skill is performed by the appropriate medical staff committee. Only then should he or she be allowed to take sole responsibility for integrating this new skill into the delivery of quality healthcare for women.

The post-graduate course should consist of didactic training (lectures and small break-out sessions) along with adequate laboratory time to perfect technical skills (Figs 1.1–1.16). Some courses may offer a live animal laboratory session, although the vast majority of the techniques may be learned using inanimate objects or extirpated animal tissue when taught at an experienced faculty. The course may be specific for hysteroscopy, operative laparoscopy (pelviscopy), or laser; often these modalities are combined into one training session for completeness. Although specific faculty members may favor one modality over another (e.g. electrocautery versus laser therapy), it is wise to learn the advantages and disadvantages of each therapy and integrate the best tips into one's particular practice.

Practice at the course and later at home, using a pelvi-trainer (Figs 1.17 and 1.18) (loaned by an instrument company, purchased by a hospital, or made by the physician), is helpful to reduce the feeling of awkwardness when performing the new surgical technique in the operating room for the first time.

Preceptorships are available with an experienced endoscopic surgeon who can supervise the preceptee during the actual operative procedure to be learned (Figs 1.19 and 1.20). The wide availability of high-resolution video cameras and monitors has facilitated closely supervised training. To maximize the preceptorship instruction, it is helpful to review the didactic material previously discussed at the prior post-graduate course before entering the operating room.

Obtaining medical staff privileges to perform the newly learned endoscopic technique is the duty of the gynecologist. Accrediting sets the minimal standards for excellence and safeguards patients, the hospital, and the physician. Documentation of post-graduate courses and preceptorships attended gives credence to the physician application. However, the hospital accrediting body is responsible for determining the individual's ability, as some physicians are limited in performing the newer techniques, in spite of attending multiple courses and/or preceptorships. For this reason, the hospital privileges may/should entail an initial number of cases to be performed under the observation of another physician, on staff, who is already accredited.

What is needed for safe operative endoscopy?

Reusable instruments

Several manufacturers distribute endoscopes with excellent viewing optics, light sources with adequate illumination for video and/or still photography, and light cables to transmit the maximum amount of light to the endoscopic field (Figs 1.21–1.49). A high-flow laparoscopic insufflator is a must for operative laparoscopy (Figs 1.50–1.53) as is a precise carbon dioxide hysteroflator for hysteroscopy (Figs 1.54 and 1.55). Laparoscopic suction-irrigators and smoke evacuators are prerequisites for the endoscopist to safely perform laser pelviscopy (Figs 1.56–1.65). Stainless steel laparoscopy and hysteroscopy instruments will enable the endoscopic surgeon to facilitate the performance of the desired technique (Figs 1.66–1.78).

Disposable instruments

Several instrument companies manufacture disposable trocars (Figs 1.79–1.91), which offer the advantages of an ever-sharp trocar coupled with a safety shield to reduce the possibility of perforating a hollow viscus upon insertion. Downsizers, to reduce the trocar opening (e.g. 10 mm to 5 mm), allow varying-sized pelviscopic instruments to be safely passed into the abdominal cavity while maintaining a satisfactory pneumoperitoneum (Figs 1.92 and 1.93). Endoscopic loops and sutures facilitate hemostasis prior to tissue removal and allow the surgeon to coapt tissue endoscopically (Figs 1.94–1.105). These endoscopic sutures may be:

(1) Endolooped to strangulate tissue to form pedicles (Figs 1.106–1.109)
(2) Sutured and tied intra-abdominally (Figs 1.110–1.120)
(3) Sutured and tied extra-corporeally (Figs 1.121–1.131)
(4) Pretied and looped sutures to be clipped or tied intra-abdominally (Figs 1.132 and 1.133)

Many disposable instruments with varying uses have been developed (Figs 1.137–1.143). The endoscopic gastrointestinal anastomosis (GIA) staples and linear cutters have greatly facilitated the ability to control hemostasis and rapidly transect vascular pedicles prior to endoscopic removal of the pathologic tissue (Figs 1.141–1.145). A hernia stapling device may be used to attach a permanent anti-adhesive barrier (Gore-Tex®) (Figs 1.146–1.152) or absorbent Interceed may be placed without stapling (Fig. 1.153). By applying FRED, an antifog aid, to the distal laparoscopic lens, condensation is reduced, thus helping to maintain a clear, unobstructed view of the surgical field (Figs 1.154–1.156).

Energy delivery systems

The most commonly used technique to maintain hemostasis is by electrocautery, either unipolar or bipolar (Figs 1.157–1.163). A good electrosurgical generator, which will produce predictable cutting and coagulating current, is essential. Thermocoagulation accomplishes tissue desiccation by electrically generating heat to 100–120°C. Although it avoids the risk of accidental electrical burn to other vital structures, its use is limited due to the time involved for heating and the possibility of accidental heat injury to other organs as the instruments slowly cool after use (Figs 1.164 and 1.165).

Lasers are able to coagulate as well as cut simultaneously, depending on the type of laser and delivery system used (Fig. 1.166). In conjunction with the laparoscope, the CO_2 laser may be delivered intra-abdominally by attaching the articulating arm directly, to a cube, or via waveguides (Figs 1.167–1.180). The fiber lasers (KTP, Argon, Nd:YAG, Diode) are less cumbersome and may be delivered by various types of flexible delivery systems (Table 1.1) (Figs 1.168–1.192). Through the hysteroscope, the Nd:YAG laser is the most powerful and the energy is delivered by bare fiber, sapphire tips, and sculpted contact tips (Figs 1.193–1.203).

Table 1.1 **Types of fiber delivery systems**			
	KTP	Argon	Nd:YAG	Diode
Bare fiber	+	+	+	+
Sculpted contact tip	+	+	+	+
Sapphire tip			+	

Photodocumentation

Small CCD (charge couple device) chip cameras have enabled the gynecologist to educate his/her patients and peers with the option of maintaining a permanent legal record (Fig. 1.204). These cameras may be directly coupled to the endoscopic lens (Figs 1.205 and 1.206), or attached via a beam-splitter which allows the surgeon to simultaneously view the operating field (Figs 1.207 and 1.208). A videotape may be made during the procedure (Fig. 1.209), or still images may be obtained optically with a Polaprint (Fig. 1.210) or by digital electronics with a Mavigraph (Fig. 1.211). A high-resolution video monitor is needed for one to work with the camera directly coupled to the endoscope. Soon the camera may be directly built into the endoscope for improved indirect video imaging of the pelvis.

35 mm Slides may be taken with the use of a 35 mm SLR (single lens reflex) camera electronically

connected to a light source with a flash generator. Although more cumbersome to use, the 35 mm format is the 'gold standard' for publication and slide presentations (Figs 1.212–1.215).

Operating room set-up

To facilitate operative endoscopic procedures, an organized approach to the multitude of technical instruments in the operating room is a must (Figs 1.216 and 1.217). Having the patient in a low lithotomy position, with the legs supported throughout (as opposed to the ankles suspended by 'candy canes'), increases access to the reproductive organs by the multiple pelviscopic instruments through the accessory puncture sites. Placing the video monitor between the patient's feet (as opposed to the patient's right side—across table) allows the surgeon to more easily work from the monitor without transposing his/her actions 90° during his/her thought processes.

Operating room team approach

It is imperative that the endoscopic surgeon is totally familiar with all the endoscopic instruments and techniques, which will reduce his/her frustrations in performing this new technique (Figs 1.218 and 1.219). It is also vital that the operating room (O.R.) scrub and circulating nurses are likewise aware, and have made sure the desired equipment is available and is in working order prior to the patient's arrival in the O.R. (Fig. 1.220). A good surgical assistant is a must, whether it be a private scrub nurse or a resident physician (Figs 1.221 and 1.222). Communication amongst the O.R. team is absolutely essential to complete the proposed surgery expeditiously. When scheduling endoscopic procedures, try to be realistic regarding the actual time needed, and relay that information as accurately as possible to the anesthesiologist and O.R. scheduling personnel. This will help prevent O.R. personnel wishing to retitle your procedures as 'horrendeoscopies' or 'everythingoscopies.'

Case selection – a rational approach to operative endoscopy

When starting out, do the easiest cases first. As your skill and confidence increase, tackle more challenging cases endoscopically. Don't forget the basic principles of hemostasis and gentle tissue handling. Keep an eye on time spent to help you decide if the patient's best interest is truly being served by not performing a laparotomy. There still remain some cases which should only be approached as an open procedure. This dilemma of operative endoscopy versus laparotomy should be decided by each individual physician based on technical skill, experience, and judgment.

Didactic training

Lectures

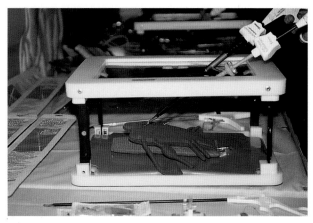

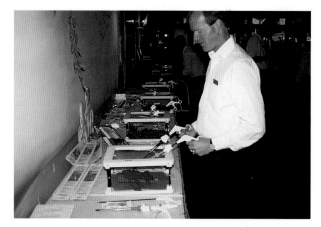

Figure 1.1 Pelvi-trainer demonstrating the use of suturing techniques on an inanimate object at the break-out session during Dr. Jack Lomano's Course on Pelviscopy at Captiva Island, April 1992.

Figure 1.2 Time is allocated at these courses to familiarize each attendee with the instrumentation and provide hands-on training prior to the actual laboratory exercises.

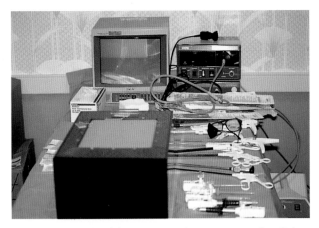

Figure 1.3 In the laboratory a video monitor with a light source and endoscopes are needed with a blackened pelvi-trainer so that the physician must focus on the video monitor to develop the necessary eye–hand coordination.

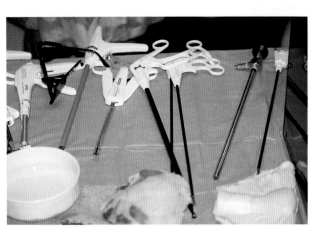

Figure 1.4 Multitude of disposable and non-disposable instruments used with a plastic model and a chicken breast.

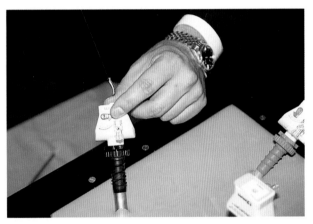

Figure 1.5 A demonstration is held to show suturing techniques by placing a disposable grasper which serves as a needle holder into the side port.

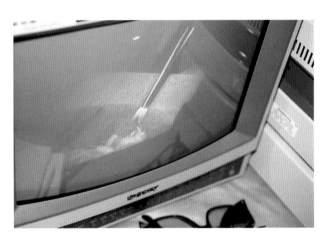

Figure 1.6 This is visualized on the video monitor as the suture is placed.

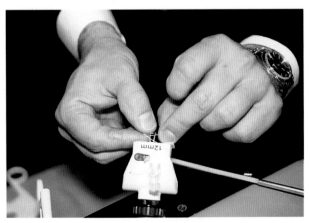

Figure 1.7 The suture is tied extra-corporeally.

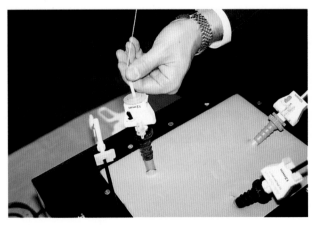

Figure 1.8 The knot is shoved along the suture to the tissue.

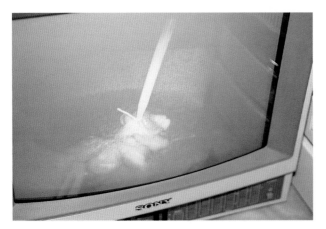

Figure 1.9 As seen on the video monitor.

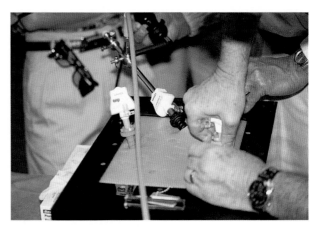

Figure 1.10 The physicians are monitored and instructed on how to place and use the disposable trocars.

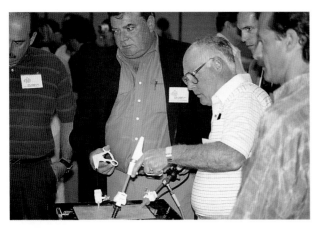

Figure 1.11 The stapling techniques are taught and practiced.

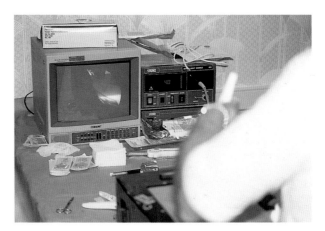

Figure 1.12 Having a video monitor enables the physician to learn how to work indirectly as well as to receive critical instruction from the faculty.

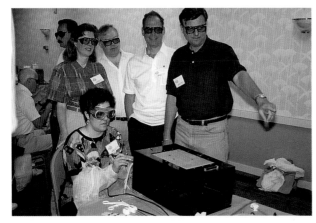

Figure 1.13 The author demonstrates to the physicians the use of the Nd:YAG laser. Note: protective eye-wear is required for all.

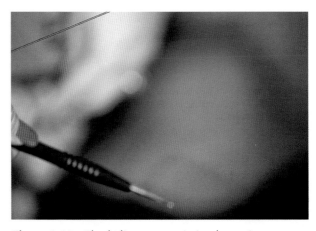

Figure 1.14 The helium–neon aiming beam is seen through the hand-held bare fiber of the Nd:YAG laser.

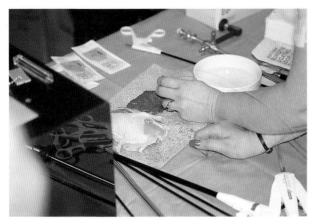

Figure 1.15 The attendees are instructed regarding the Nd:YAG laser tissue effects on liver and chicken breasts, with a high absorption of the laser energy by the darkened liver.

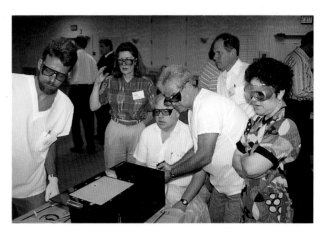

Figure 1.16 Dr. Jack Lomano instructs the use of the Nd:YAG laser hysteroscopically in a cow uterus.

Practice

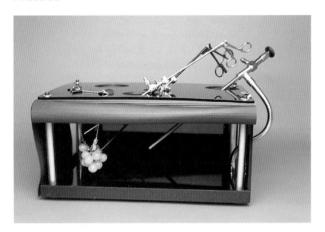

Figure 1.17 The pelvi-trainer may be purchased from Storz to use at home or hospital (courtesy of Storz).

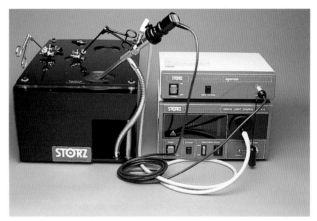

Figure 1.18 Attached to a light source with a video camera, the pelvi-trainer enables the learning pelviscopic surgeon to develop his/her technique (courtesy of Storz).

Preceptorship

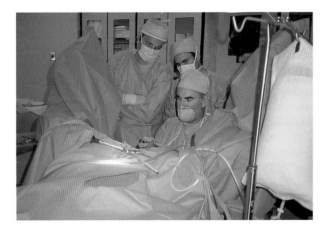

Figure 1.19 Preceptorships are available with faculty members, as seen with Dr. Jim Daniell in Nashville, Tennessee.

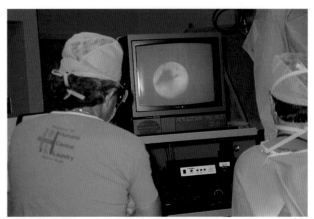

Figure 1.20 Having a video monitor enables the preceptee to observe the proper technique of endometrial ablation with the author.

Instruments

Reusable

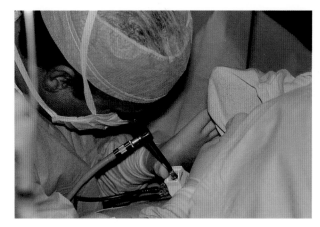

Figure 1.21 Laparoscopy for diagnostic and operative purposes is best accomplished using a 10 mm laparoscope for the expanded operative field.

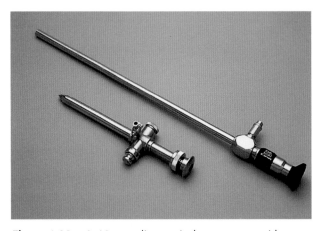

Figure 1.22 A 10 mm diagnostic laparoscope with trocar sheath (courtesy of Storz).

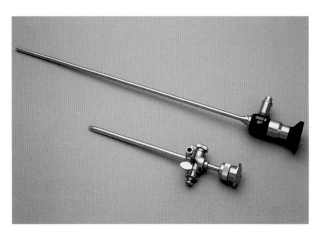

Figure 1.23 A 5 mm diagnostic laparoscope with trocar sheath (courtesy of Storz).

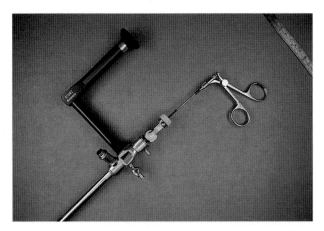

Figure 1.24 The 12 mm operative laparoscope consists of a 5 mm viewing channel and an 8 mm operating channel which enables instruments to be passed through the single-puncture scope or a laser to be attached.

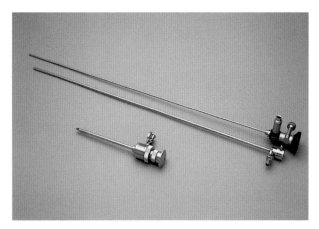

Figure 1.25 A 3 mm tuboscope with a sleeve through which CO_2 may be insufflated to dilate the fimbria from a second-puncture 5 mm trocar (courtesy of Storz).

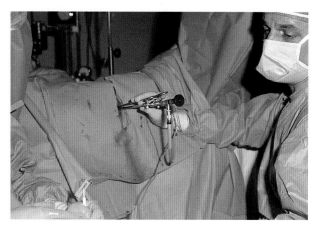

Figure 1.26 Hysteroscopy may be diagnostic or operative.

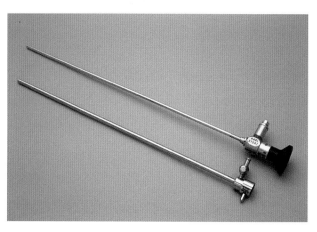

Figure 1.27 A 3 mm diagnostic hysteroscope (courtesy of Storz).

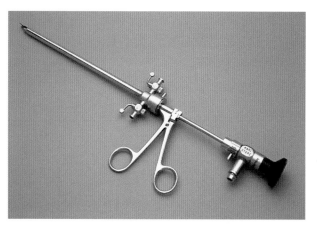

Figure 1.28 A rigid operative hysteroscope—assembled (courtesy of Storz).

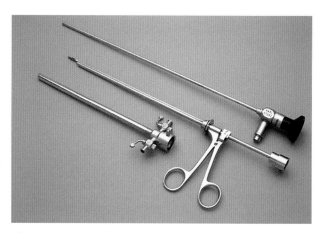

Figure 1.29 Rigid operative hysteroscope disassembled. Note the scissors on the middle sheath for accomplishing a transcervical metroplasty (courtesy of Storz).

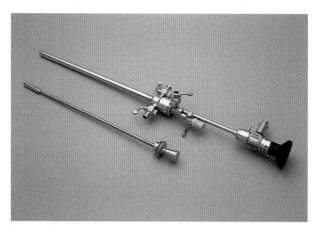

Figure 1.30 Laser hysteroscope having a constant flow-through channel with a port for the laser fiber, along with an introducing trocar (courtesy of Storz).

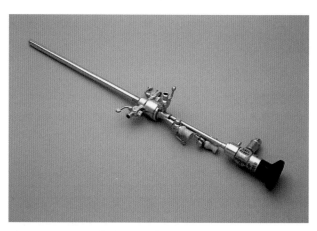

Figure 1.31 Dual-channel laser hysteroscope allowing for suction (courtesy of Storz).

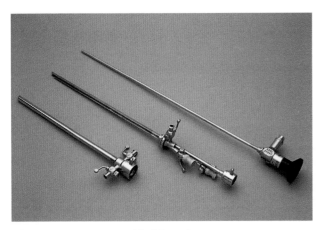

Figure 1.32 Disassembled laser hysteroscope (courtesy of Storz).

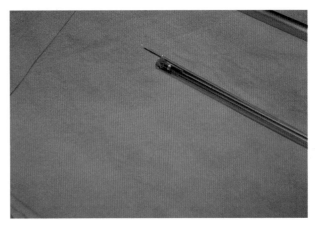

Figure 1.33 Bare Nd:YAG fiber seen at the tip of the hysteroscope.

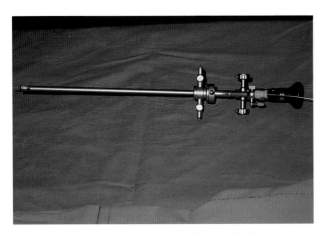

Figure 1.34 Hysteroscope with Albarran bridge.

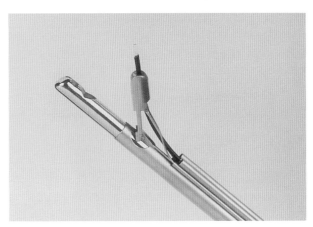

Figure 1.35 The Albarran bridge hinges at the tip of the scope which is controlled by the knurled knobs adjacent to the eyepiece.

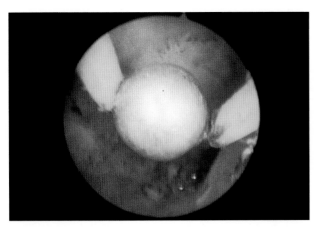

Figure 1.36 Operative resectoscope as viewed with the rollerball.

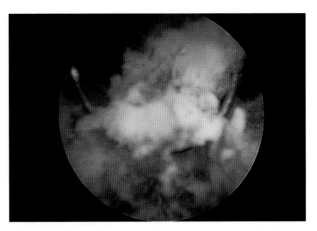

Figure 1.37 Operative resectoscope as seen with the electrical loop.

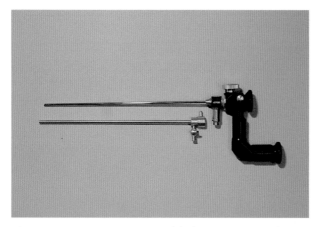

Figure 1.38 Hamou micro-colpo hysteroscope with sheath. This consists of a 3 mm diagnostic hysteroscope with multiple magnifications. Panoramic and contact views of tissue pathology in the fundus of the uterus and endocervix are possible.

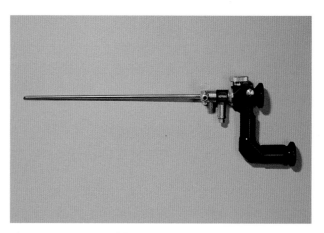

Figure 1.39 Assembled Hamou hysteroscope.

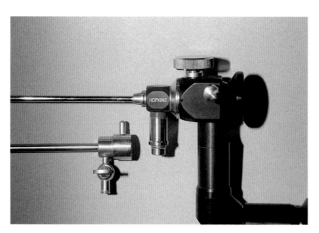

Figure 1.40 Close-up of the focusing knob for the hysteroscope. This device is excellent for diagnostic hysteroscopy in the office setting as it may be passed without dilatation into the multiparous cervix.

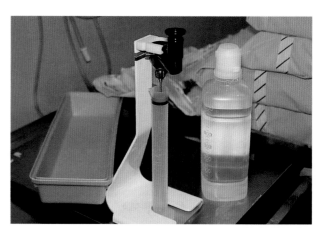

Figure 1.41 Unfortunately the eyepiece of the hysteroscope cannot be soaked, thus the tip needs to be placed in cidex and rinsed prior to use.

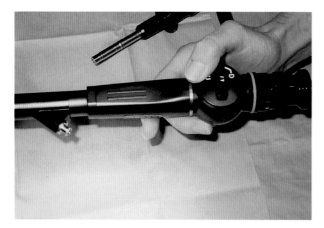

Figure 1.42 The steering control seen with the Olympus flexible hysteroscope.

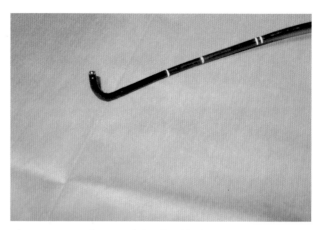

Figure 1.43 The tip of the flexible hysteroscope.

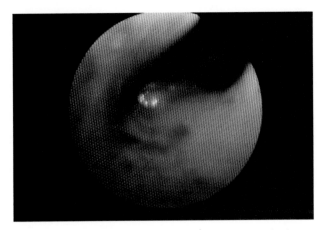

Figure 1.44 A view through the hysteroscope which facilitates seeing into the cornua.

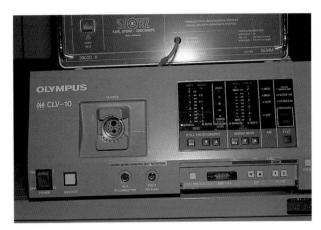

Figure 1.45 Olympus video light source allowing videotaping and still photography with its built-in electronic flash.

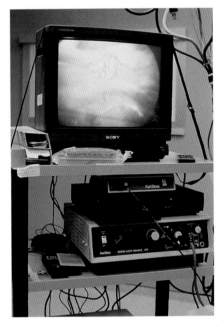

Figure 1.46 Storz light source and video monitor.

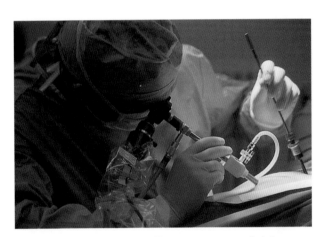

Figure 1.47 Appropriate illumination is needed for videotaping the laparoscopic procedure.

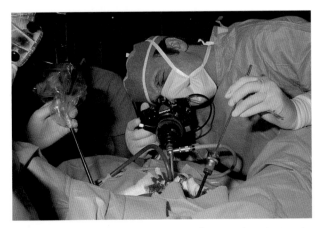

Figure 1.48 35 mm Still photography may be obtained by using electronic flash.

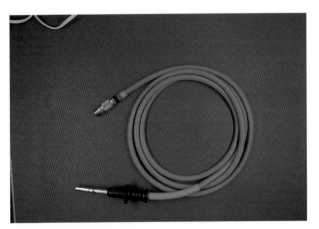

Figure 1.49 A fiber-optic cable in good condition is vital to appropriate illumination for photography. Care must be taken to avoid breaking the fibers; the cable should be checked frequently to avoid shadows and hot spots.

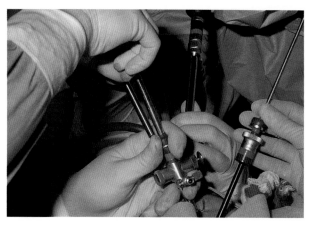

Figure 1.50 Multiple punctures through the abdominal wall with pelviscopy affords the opportunity for CO_2 gas leakage requiring a high-flow insufflator.

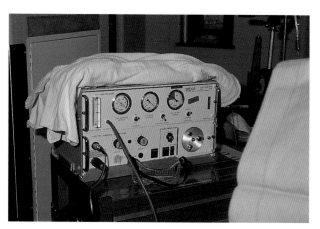

Figure 1.51 Standard non-electronic laparoscopic insufflators control the gas flow at one liter to three liters per minute.

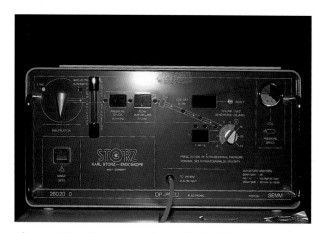

Figure 1.52 The newer electronic insufflators provide flow up to seven liters per minute.

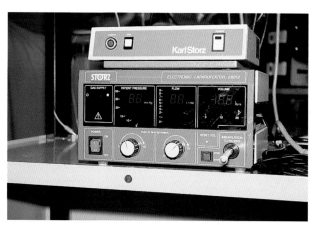

Figure 1.53 The newest model of the Storz electronic insufflator is more compact (courtesy of Storz).

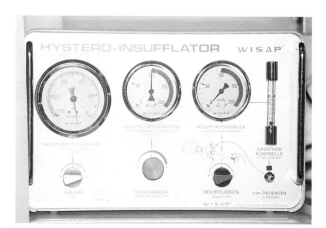

Figure 1.54 The hystero-insufflator for hysteroscopy should not exceed 100 ml per minute which is controlled by manual settings.

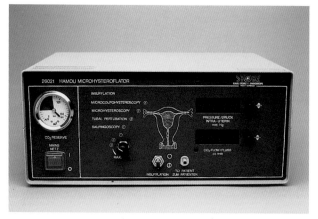

Figure 1.55 Electronic monitoring of the hysteroscopic flow is afforded by the newer hystero-insufflator (courtesy of Storz).

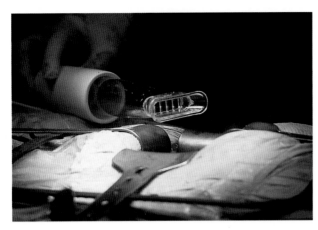

Figure 1.56 At open laparotomy a suction device is needed to reduce the toxic laser smoke. It is vital to place the suction tip close to the abdominal wound to capture the smoke as soon as it exits the abdominal cavity.

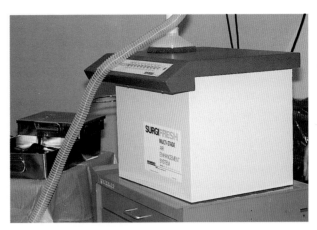

Figure 1.57 The laser suction device should be able to filter to 0.1 micron in order to trap the carbon particles in laser smoke.

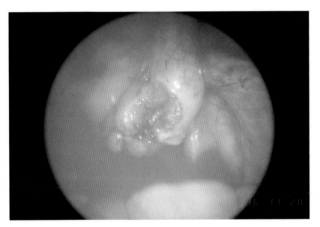

Figure 1.58 A laparoscopic view of laser laparoscopic neosalpingostomy shows marked smoke accumulation using the CO_2 laser.

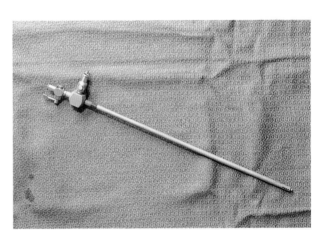

Figure 1.59 A suction-irrigation probe should be used to help evacuate the smoke.

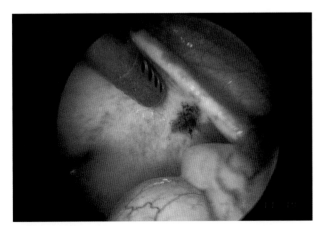

Figure 1.60 The tip of the suction-irrigator should be placed close to the lesion to be lasered in order to capture the smoke as soon as possible and avoid circulating the gas through the abdominal cavity.

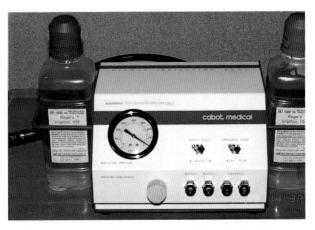

Figure 1.61 Aqua-dissection is useful to hydro-dissect densely coapted tissue.

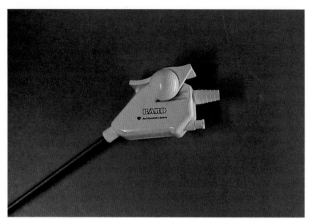

Figure 1.62 Disposable suction-irrigator from Bard allows fingertip control for profuse irrigation and suction which is often required for ruptured ectopic pregnancies.

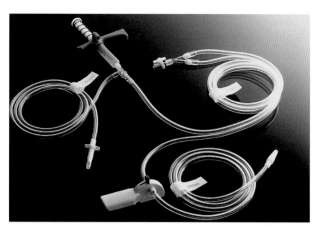

Figure 1.63 A photograph of the new Pump Vac III valve which allows fingertip control of irrigation of suction (courtesy of Marlow Surgical Technologies).

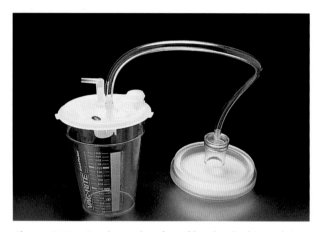

Figure 1.64 Smoke and carbon filter hooked into the plastic liquid reservoir to allow for a concomitant suction irrigation (courtesy of Surgi-Medics).

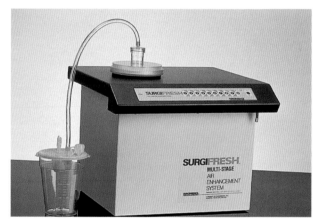

Figure 1.65 Suction device with the canisters and filters attached (courtesy of Surgi-Medics).

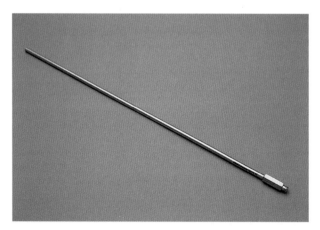

Figure 1.66 A 5 mm probe is the most useful instrument for diagnostic laparoscopy (courtesy of Storz).

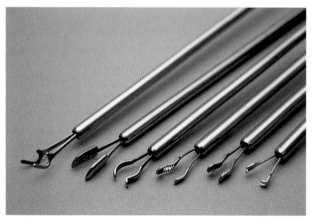

Figure 1.67 A multitude of non-disposable stainless steel graspers (courtesy of Storz).

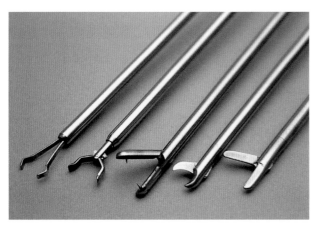

Figure 1.68 There are also a multitude of hook scissors with coagulators and graspers available (courtesy of Storz).

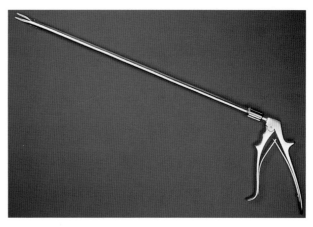

Figure 1.69 A non-disposable clip applicator.

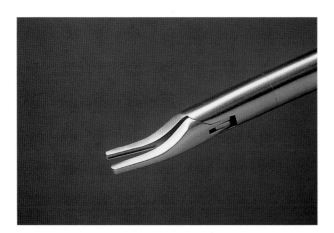

Figure 1.70 A close-up of the clip applicator.

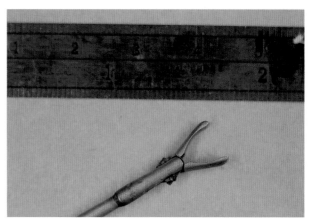

Figure 1.71 A 3 mm grasper is atraumatic and particularly useful for grasping fimbria for GIFT procedures.

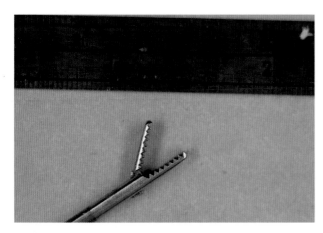

Figure 1.72 A 3 mm needle holder for pelviscopic suturing.

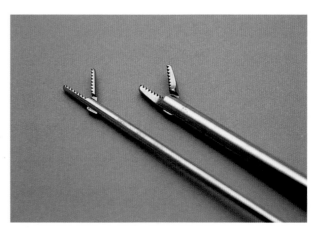

Figure 1.73 The 3 mm and 5 mm needle holders (courtesy of Storz).

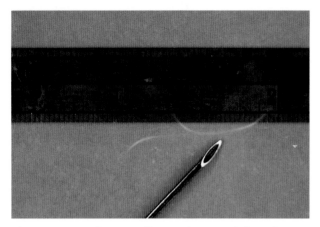

Figure 1.74 A long needle may be passed through a 3 mm or 5 mm port, in order to decompress ovarian cysts.

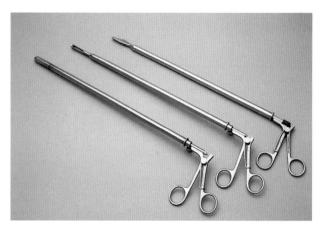

Figure 1.75 10 mm Instruments are useful to grasp and cut tissue such as fibroids and ectopics. These are passed through the umbilical port with a 5 mm laparoscope placed through the second puncture for observation (courtesy of Storz).

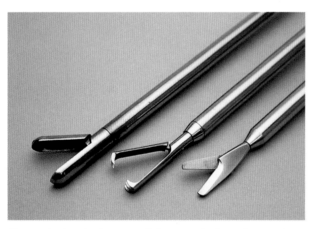

Figure 1.76 A close-up of the cup device, claw and scissors (courtesy of Storz).

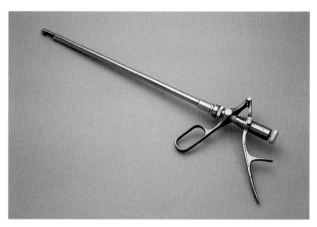

Figure 1.77 A morcellator is helpful to bite pieces of tissue and remove fibroids (courtesy of Storz).

Disposable trocars

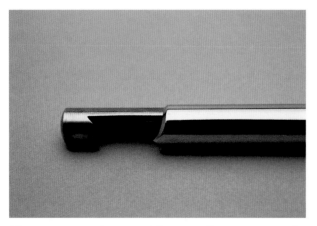

Figure 1.78 A close-up of the morcellator (courtesy of Storz).

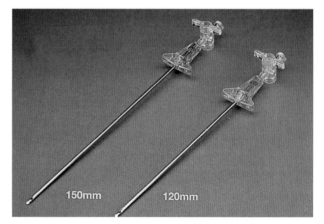

Figure 1.79 Disposable Verres needles are helpful particularly in the 150 mm length for obese patients in establishing a pneumoperitoneum (courtesy of U.S. Surgical Corporation).

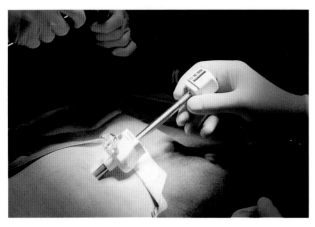

Figure 1.80 Disposable trocars usually provide a safe entrance into the abdominal cavity.

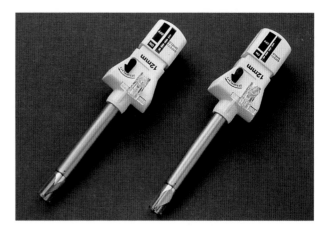

Figure 1.81 A 12 mm U.S. Surgical trocar (courtesy of U.S. Surgical).

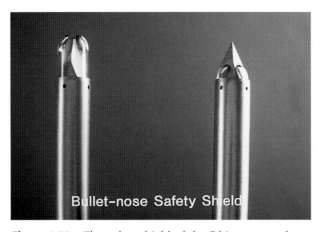

Figure 1.82 The safety shield of the Ethicon trocar has a rounded tip facilitating placement into the tissue (courtesy of Ethicon).

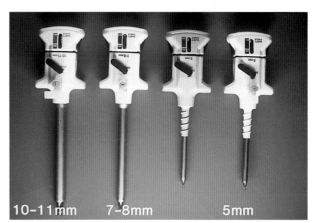

Figure 1.83 The trocars come in varying sizes (courtesy of Ethicon).

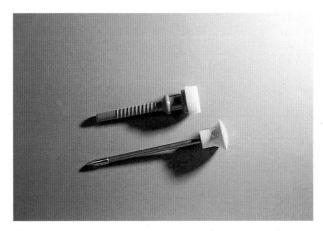

Figure 1.84 A short 5 mm trocar with an external screw design made by Apple is an excellent second-puncture trocar.

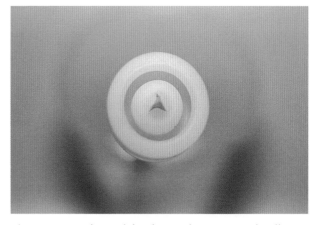

Figure 1.85 The seal for the Apple trocar easily allows 5 mm or 3 mm instruments to be passed without a downsizer due to its design.

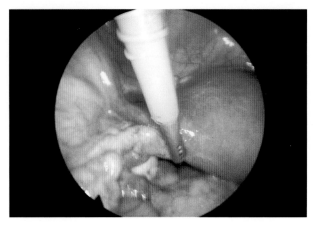

Figure 1.86 The external screw pattern fixes the trocar through the fascia to facilitate the passing of the instruments.

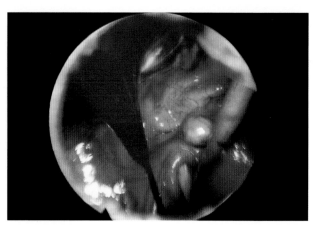

Figure 1.87 If an abdominal wall bleeder is found, Marlow has devised a trocar to apply pressure from within the abdominal wall as well as externally compressing the abdominal wall to control the bleeding.

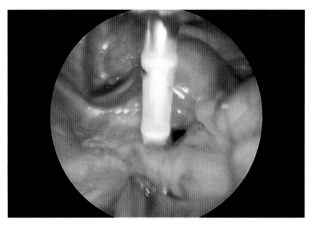

Figure 1.88 The trocar has a balloon similar to a Foley bulb which is decompressed as the trocar is inserted.

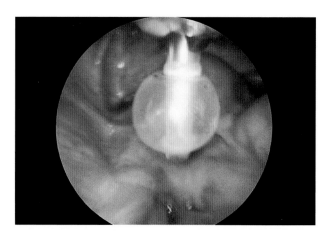

Figure 1.89 The bulb is inflated through an external port.

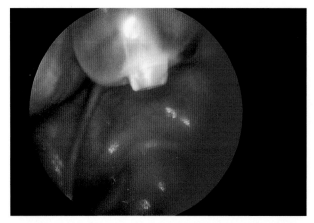

Figure 1.90 The bulb is withdrawn toward the abdominal wall and pressure is applied from an external ring.

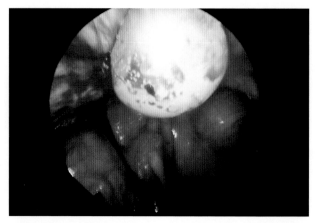

Figure 1.91 The bleeding is controlled through a 5 mm channel; an instrument may still be passed enabling the laparoscopist to continue his/her procedure.

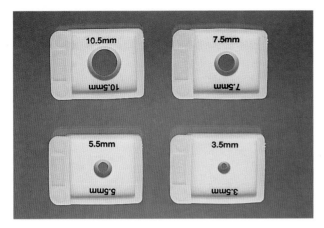

Figure 1.92 Downsizers are used to reduce the port size for varying instruments. Thus a 10 mm trocar may be used and downsized for a 3 mm instrument and still retain the pneumoperitoneum (courtesy of U.S. Surgical).

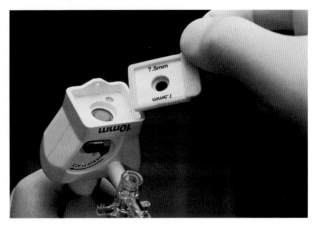

Figure 1.93 A 7.5 mm downsizer is being placed into the 10 mm trocar (courtesy of U.S. Surgical).

Endoscopic sutures

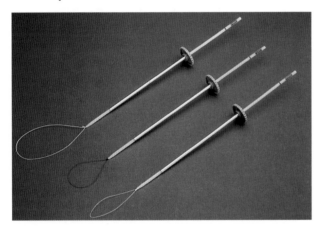

Figure 1.94 Loop ligatures are available in PDS, Vicryl and chromic to allow for snaring tissue. They may come within their own passer to facilitate introduction through the trocar valve (courtesy of U.S. Surgical).

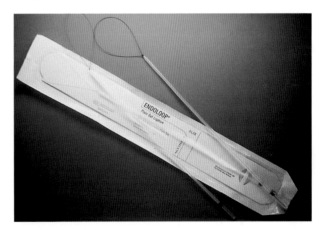

Figure 1.95 Endoloops were first devised by Ethicon to snare and strangulate the tissue.

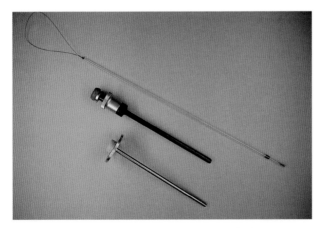

Figure 1.96 The endoloop should be loaded into a passer in order to avoid the trocar trap.

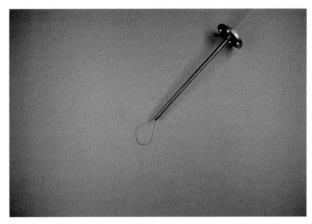

Figure 1.97 The endoloop backloaded into the passer device.

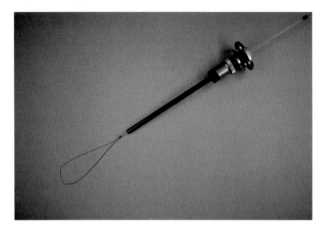

Figure 1.98 The endoloop and passer placed through the trocar.

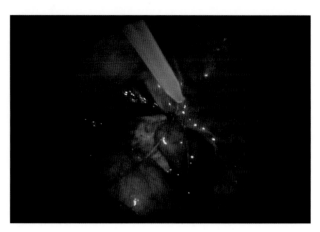

Figure 1.99 The tissue is strangulated and the knot pusher forces the knot down.

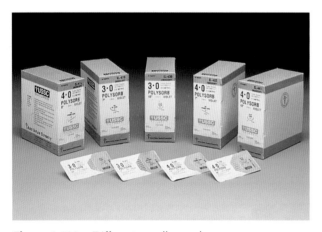

Figure 1.100 Different needles and sutures are available (courtesy of U.S. Surgical).

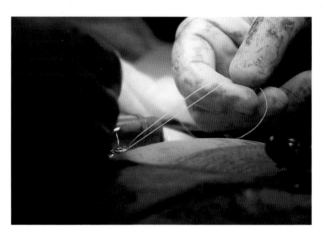

Figure 1.101 The knot may be tied extra-corporeally as seen here or intra-abdominally.

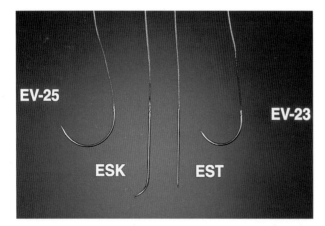

Figure 1.102 Needles are available in hooked, curved, and a ski tip facilitating placement into the tissue (courtesy of U.S. Surgical).

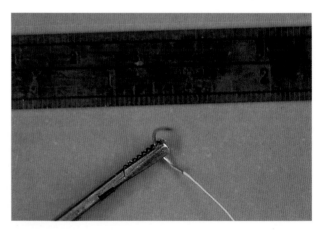

Figure 1.103 The needle holder grasps the curved needle on a flat portion of the needle.

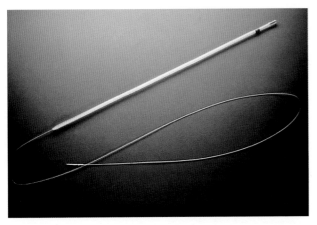

Figure 1.104 Needles with a knot pusher are available for extra-corporeal knot tying (courtesy of U.S. Surgical).

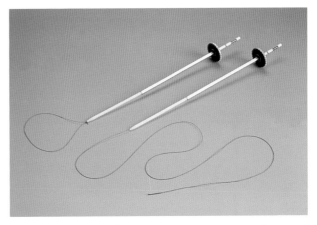

Figure 1.105 Needles with a knot pusher are also available with their own passers for placement through the trocars (courtesy of U.S. Surgical).

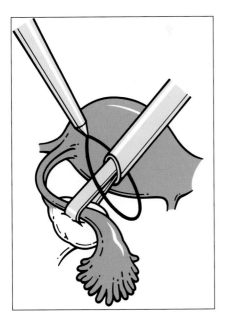

Figure 1.106 An endoloop is placed over a grasper prior to grabbing the left tube and ovary.

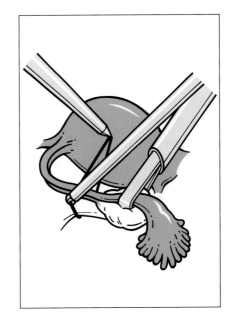

Figure 1.107 The endoloop is placed at the base of the vascular pedicle and snugged down.

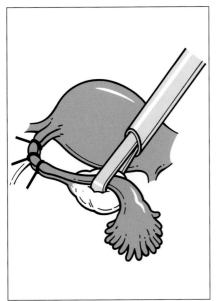

Figure 1.108 Three endoloops have been placed to strangulate the blood supply to the left adnexa.

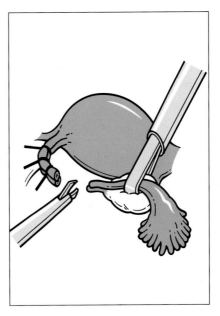

Figure 1.109 Scissors excise the tube and ovary.

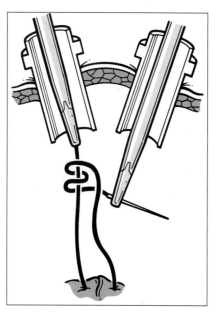

Figure 1.110
A Roeder loop is initiated endoscopically by making a half-hitch.

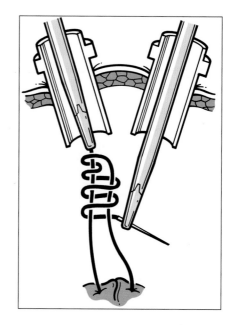

Figure 1.111
The suture is wound about *both* suture arms times three.

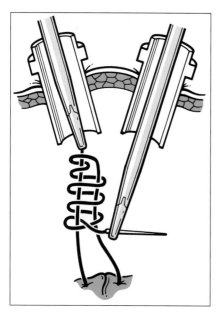

Figure 1.112
The knot is finished by another half-hitch around the initial arm.

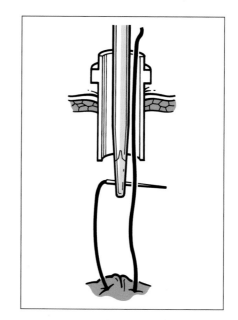

Figure 1.113
A fisherman's clinch knot is initiated by placing the straight needle perpendicular to the initial arm of the suture.

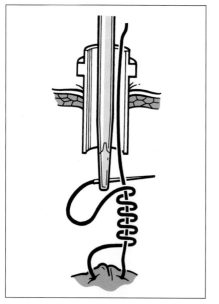

Figure 1.114
The needle is spun several times (×5).

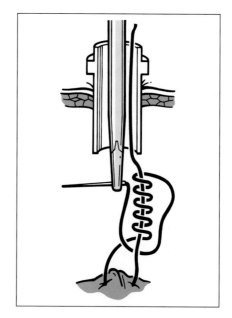

Figure 1.115
The needle is brought between the tissue and initial loop and tightened.

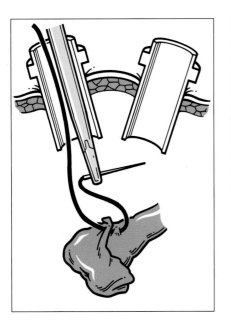

Figure 1.116
Intra-abdominal knot tying begins by suturing the two tissue leaves together, then removing the needle.

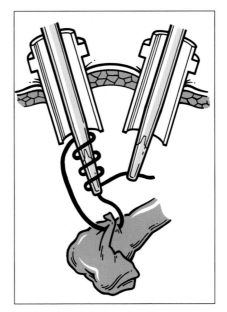

Figure 1.117
The initial needle holder begins an endoscopic instrument tie by wrapping the long arm of the suture about itself.

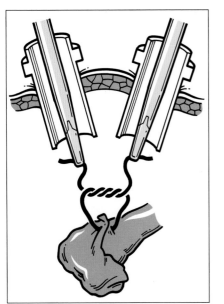

Figure 1.118
Each needle holder pulls the arms of the suture to lay down a flat double-throw surgeon's knot.

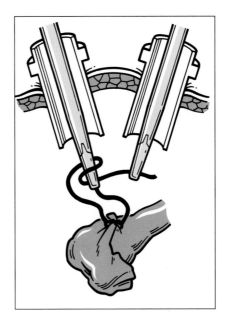

Figure 1.119
The second instrument tie is accomplished.

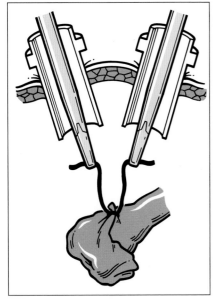

Figure 1.120
A square knot is the final result.

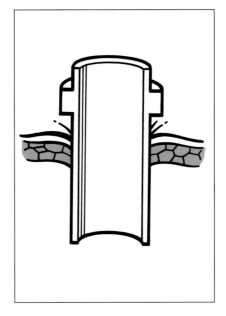

Figure 1.121
A short trocar is placed in the lower abdomen.

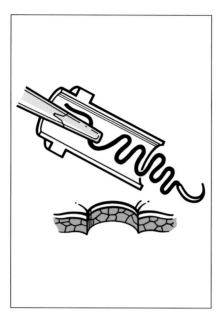

Figure 1.122
The suture is backloaded into the trocar with the sleeve withdrawn from the abdomen.

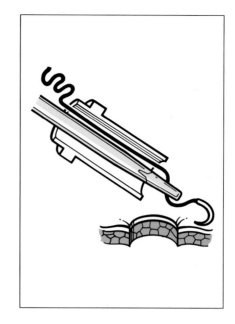

Figure 1.123
The suture is grasped by the needle holder about 3 cm from the base of the curved needle.

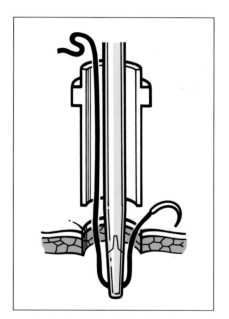

Figure 1.124
The needle holder is placed through the abdominal puncture wound.

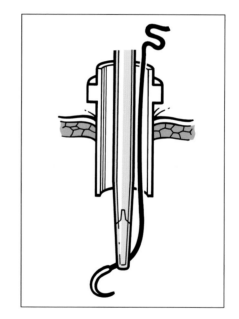

Figure 1.125
The sleeve is replaced through the abdominal wall over the needle holder.

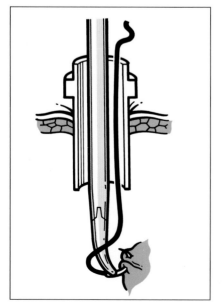

Figure 1.126
The needle is grasped by the needle holder and the tissue leaves are sutured together.

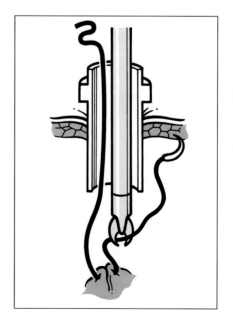

Figure 1.127
The needle is attached to the anterior abdominal wall, and the suture cut about 3 cm from the needle.

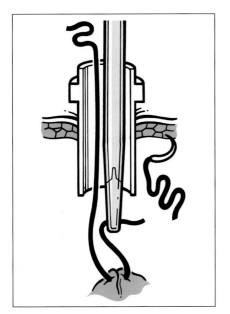

Figure 1.128
The short arm of the suture is brought through the trocar extra-abdominally for an extra-corporeal tie.

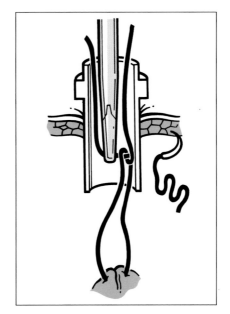

Figure 1.129
The extra-corporeal knot is laid down by the needle holder or a knot pusher.

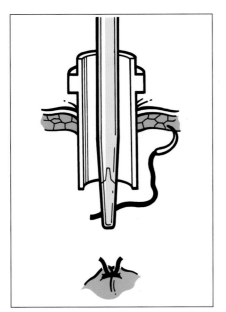

Figure 1.130
The needle is retrieved.

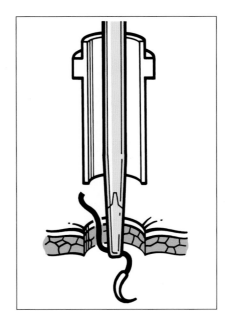

Figure 1.131
The needle is brought out after the trocar sleeve is removed.

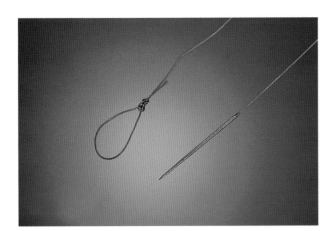

Figure 1.132   A short pre-tied loop of suture with a needle is also available to facilitate intra-abdominal suturing and tying by placing a clip to complete the knot tying (courtesy of U.S. Surgical).

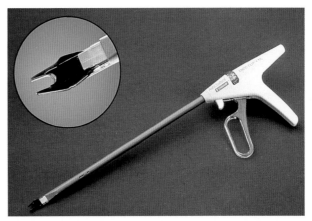

Figure 1.133   An endoscopic clip may be placed on the suture after the needle has been passed through the pre-tied loop for tissue fixation.

Disposable laparoscopic instruments

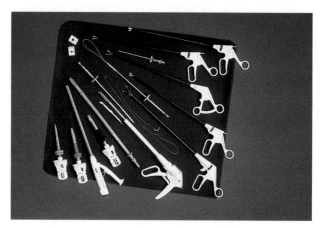

Figure 1.134 Multiple disposable instruments are available (courtesy of U.S. Surgical).

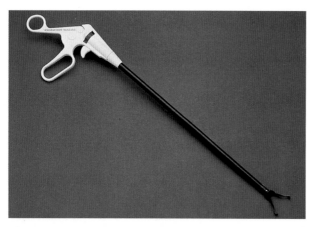

Figure 1.135 A 10 mm grasper is used to hold the ovary (courtesy of U.S. Surgical).

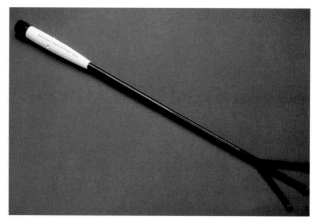

Figure 1.136 An endoretractor is useful to withdraw tissue through the surgical port (courtesy of U.S. Surgical).

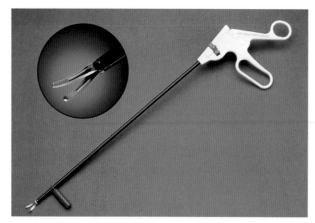

Figure 1.137 Endoscopic Metzenbaum scissors are used for tissue dissection and may be locked into place and double as a needle holder (courtesy of U.S. Surgical).

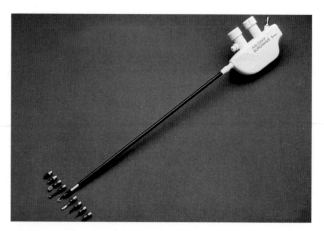

Figure 1.138 Disposable electrocautery devices with multiple tips may be helpful as well (courtesy of U.S. Surgical).

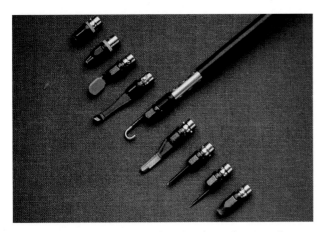

Figure 1.139 Note the multitude of tips for unipolar cautery (courtesy of U.S. Surgical).

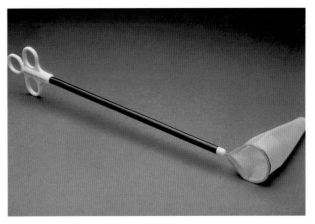

Figure 1.140 A specimen bag is available to facilitate tissue removal (courtesy of U.S. Surgical).

Endoscopic GIA, staplers, and linear cutters

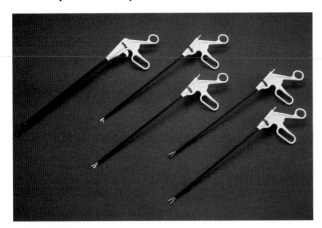

Figure 1.141 A multitude of stapling devices have been developed to facilitate hemostasis and cutting in one action (courtesy of U.S. Surgical).

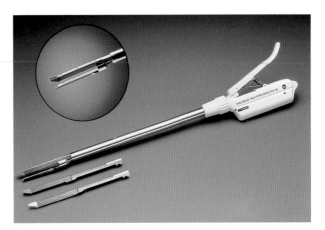

Figure 1.142 The single-fire endoscopic gastrointestinal anastomosis (GIA) is placed through a large port to grasp the tissue and cut it (courtesy of U.S. Surgical).

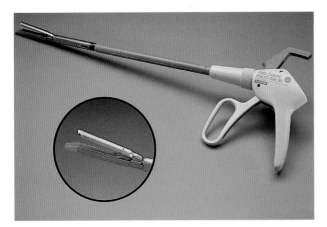

Figure 1.143 A multi-fire endoscopic GIA may be used up to four times for a similar purpose. The top gray handle is used to open the device prior to clamping the tissue (courtesy of U.S. Surgical).

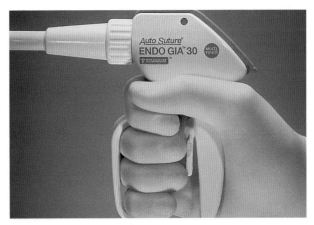

Figure 1.144 The gray handle is closed to grasp the tissue then the device is fired by squeezing the pistol grip. The tissue is then released by opening the gray lever (courtesy of U.S. Surgical).

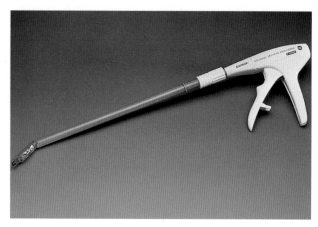

Figure 1.145 In order to assess tissue thickness to determine which stapling cartridge is needed, a measuring device is first placed over the tissue (courtesy of U.S. Surgical).

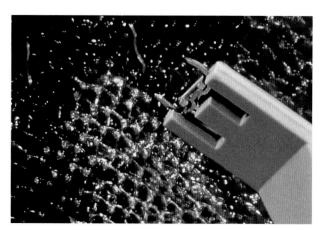

Figure 1.146 The endoscopic hernia stapling device has an angled head (courtesy of U.S. Surgical).

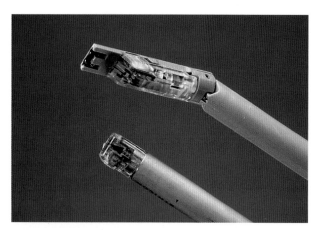

Figure 1.147 A close-up view of the stapling mechanism (courtesy of U.S. Surgical).

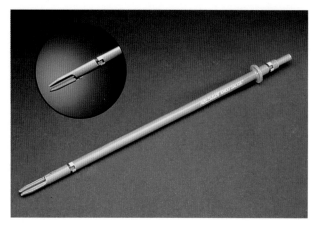

Figure 1.148 This device enables the placement of a mesh over the hernia defect (courtesy of U.S. Surgical).

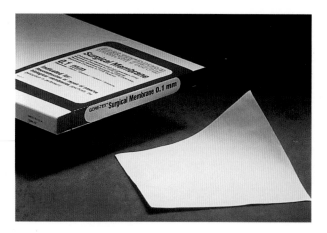

Figure 1.149 In gynecological pelviscopy, this device is also quite helpful to place a Gore-Tex® patch over a denuded peritoneal surface in an effort to prevent adhesion reformation (courtesy of W.L. Gore).

Adhesive barriers

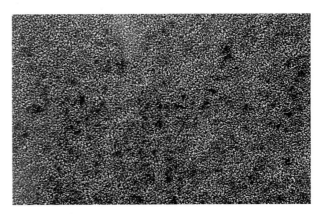

Figure 1.150   A scanning electron micrograph (SEM) of the surgical membrane, showing the microstructure of the Gore-Tex® patch connected with fibrils (courtesy of W.L. Gore).

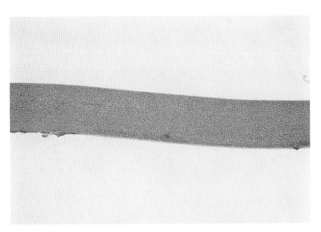

Figure 1.151   Histology of a retrieved Gore-Tex® surgical membrane from its previously used site; note that no adhesions are attached to either side of the membrane (courtesy of W.L. Gore).

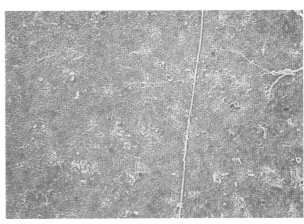

Figure 1.152   A SEM of the surgical membrane after four years of attachment over a myomectomy incision. Note how it appears similar to the previous SEM slide showing no tissue reactivity (courtesy of W.L. Gore).

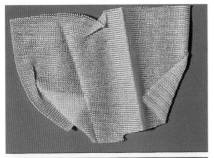

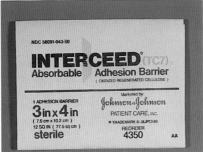

Figure 1.153   Interceed may also be used, which is an absorbable adhesion barrier devised by Johnson & Johnson. This is a chemically-enhanced form of surgicel which may be used in non-hemorrhagic areas and is usually absorbed at the end of the six-week healing process.

Defogging devices

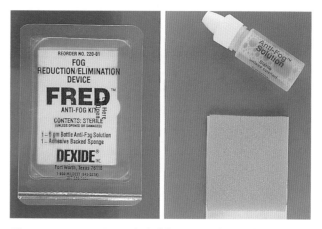

Figure 1.154 FRED is helpful to coat the endoscopic lens to allow clear viewing by preventing fogging.

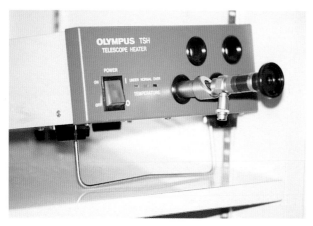

Figure 1.155 A telescopic heater made by Olympus will warm the scopes in an effort to reduce fogging.

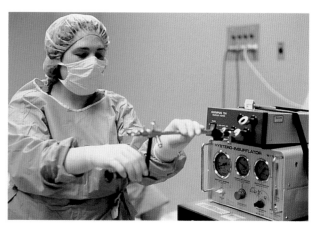

Figure 1.156 Multiple endoscopes may be placed and retrieved as needed.

Electrocautery

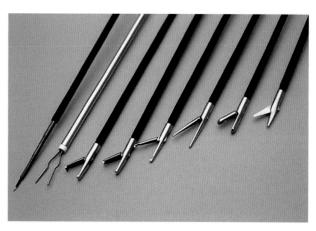

Figure 1.157 Different cautery tips are available in non-disposable instruments (courtesy of Storz).

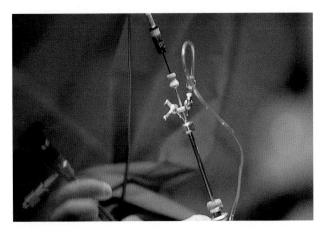

Figure 1.158 The micro-cautery with a suction-irrigation port (5 mm) is quite helpful to endoscopically control small bleeders.

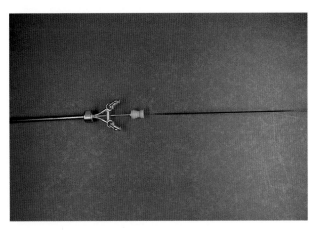

Figure 1.159 The electrode is placed through a rubber cap into the central port.

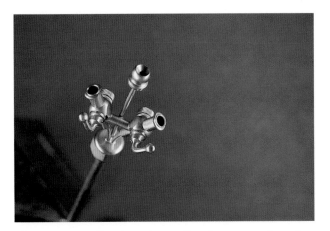

Figure 1.160 The three ports allow for connection of irrigation and suction.

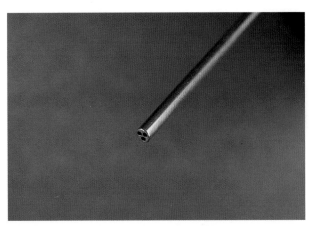

Figure 1.161 The suction port is not helpful for massive withdrawal of fluids but is helpful to control small bleeders. The maximum power to be used should be restricted to 20 watts to avoid burning the tip of the electrode.

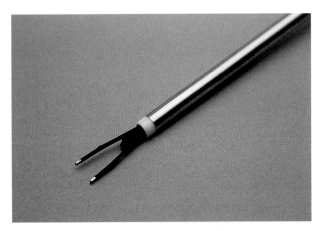

Figure 1.162 Bipolar cautery is helpful for spot bleeders (courtesy of Storz).

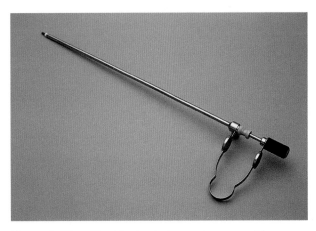

Figure 1.163 The bipolar instrument comes with a spring grip handle (courtesy of Storz).

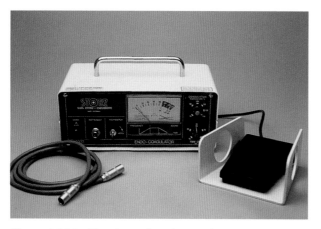

Figure 1.164 The thermal endocoagulator energy source (courtesy of Storz).

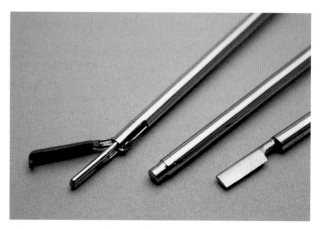

Figure 1.165 Endocoagulator instruments which heat up and have no electrical charge (courtesy of Storz).

Lasers

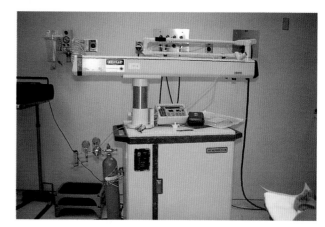

Figure 1.166 A Sharplan 1100 CO_2 laser generates 100 watts of CO_2 laser energy with 35 watts of superpulse.

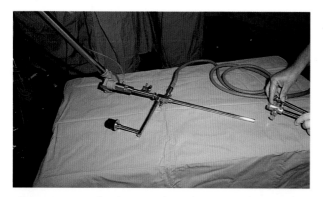

Figure 1.167 The first CO_2 laparoscope used in North America in 1980 by Dr. Jim Daniel was a modified Eder bronchoscope connected directly to the articulating arm of a 733 Sharplan laser. A marked amount of time was needed to reflect the beam directly through the 5 mm operating channel.

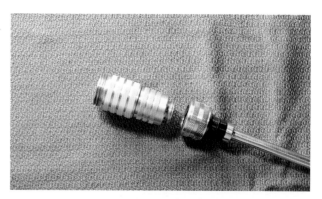

Figure 1.168 A 425 mm laser lens was attached to a sheath with an 8 mm operating channel enabling the author to perform second-puncture CO_2 laser laparoscopy in 1981.

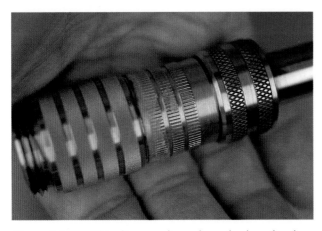

Figure 1.169 This diagram shows how the lens fits the operating sheath.

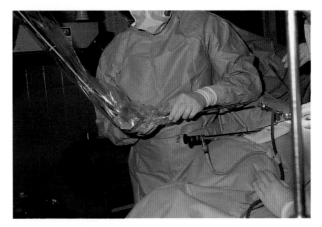

Figure 1.170 The operating sheath is attached to the articulating arm of the CO_2 laser.

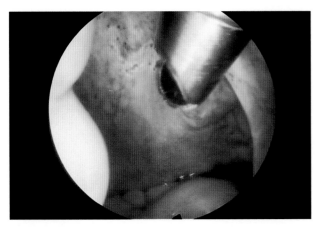

Figure 1.171 A 45° mirror is used at the tip of the sheath to enable the CO_2 laser beam to attack the tissue at a 90° angle.

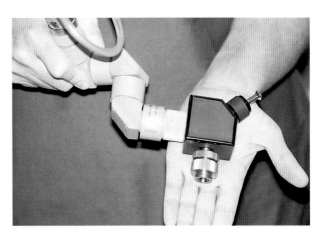

Figure 1.172 In 1983, the Eder cube was developed which allowed for a gimbaled mirror to guide the He–Ne beam and subsequently the CO_2 laser beam into the center of the operating channel.

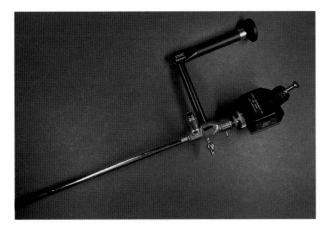

Figure 1.173 This diagram shows the Eder cube attached to the Storz operating laparoscope with its 8 mm operating channel.

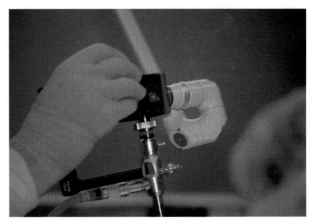

Figure 1.174 Usually an outer glove is placed to facilitate centering the beam through the operating channel and then the glove is discarded.

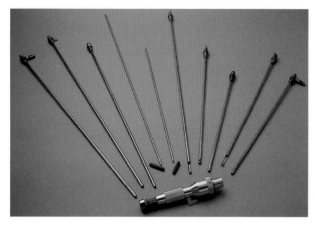

Figure 1.175 Sharplan wave guides were developed which help to overcome the misaligned articulating arm of the CO_2 laser and facilitate second-puncture laser laparoscopy (courtesy of Sharplan).

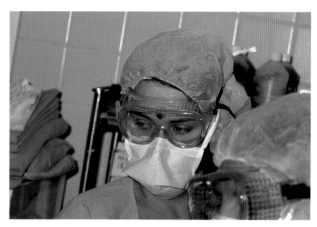

Figure 1.176 With CO_2 laser energy in the room, the operating room personnel are required to wear clear glasses.

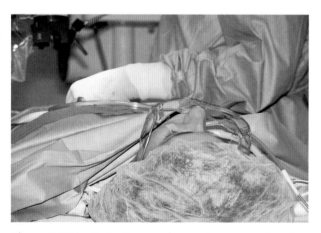

Figure 1.177 Protective goggles or glasses are placed over the patient.

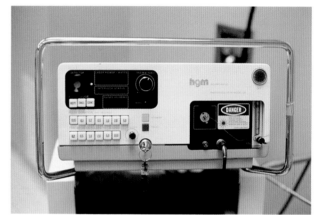

Figure 1.178 The 12 watt HGM argon laser.

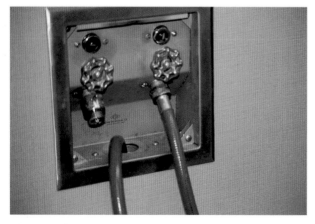

Figure 1.179 An external circulating water source is required for cooling, along with 220 volt electrical service for most of the fiber lasers.

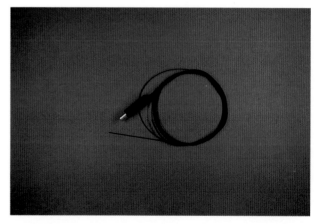

Figure 1.180 The advantage of the argon laser is its ability to be delivered through a flexible fiber.

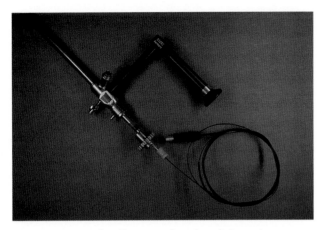

Figure 1.181 This fiber may be placed through a single-puncture laparoscope and, by adjusting the knurled knob, directed to the tissue.

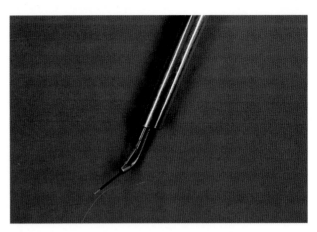

Figure 1.182 The tip of the fiber director.

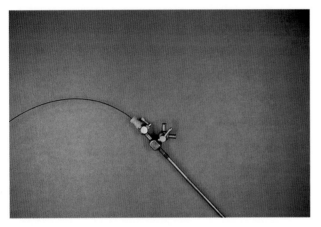

Figure 1.183 The author prefers to use the fiber through a second puncture in order to have a better sense of depth perception. This second-puncture fiber probe has a suction–irrigation channel as well.

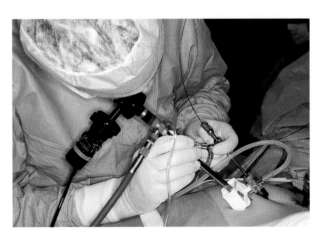

Figure 1.184 The fiber being used through the second puncture.

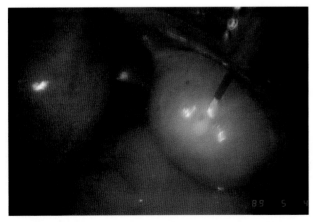

Figure 1.185 A visible blue-green light is seen through the bar argon fiber.

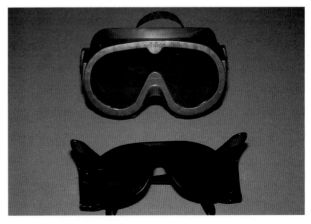

Figure 1.186 Orange-colored goggles or glasses are required to protect the retina of the operating room personnel.

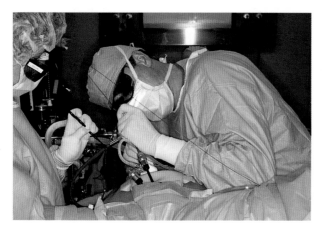

Figure 1.187 Protective eyewear is required to protect the eyes of the surgeon.

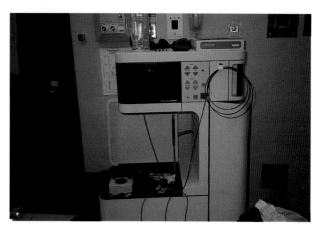

Figure 1.188 The KTP laser has a similar tissue effect as the argon laser and also requires modification of the operating room for electrical and plumbing service.

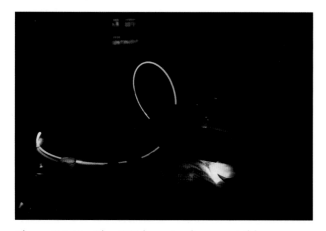

Figure 1.189 The KTP laser produces a visible green light (courtesy of Laserscope).

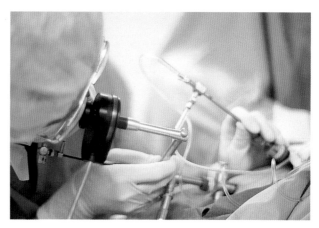

Figure 1.190 There is an optical filter that is placed over the eyepiece to protect the surgeon's retina and is activated by depressing the foot pedal (courtesy of Jim Daniell, M.D.).

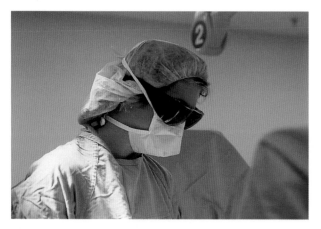

Figure 1.191 The O.R. personnel are required to wear protective glasses or goggles to avoid retinal damage.

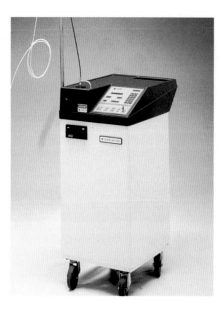

Figure 1.192 The Sharplan Nd:YAG laser.

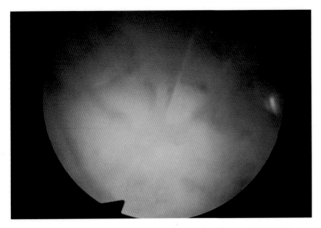

Figure 1.193 Hysteroscopic view of a bare Nd:YAG fiber.

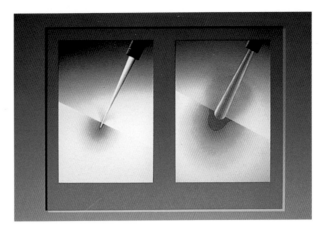

Figure 1.194 With a non-contact bare fiber, forward scatter as well as back scatter occurs, which is useful for endometrial ablation. Using a sapphire tip, the fiber may be placed in contact with the tissue and the tissue effect limited (courtesy of SLT).

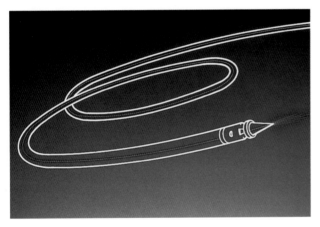

Figure 1.195 The sapphire tip heats up to obtain the required tissue effect (courtesy of SLT).

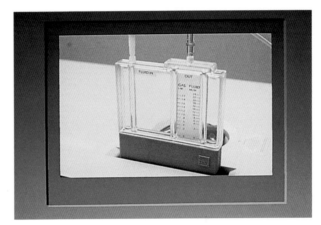

Figure 1.196 The tips need to be cooled either by CO_2 or fluid when used laparoscopically, but should *not* be used hysteroscopically due to the risk of air embolus (courtesy of SLT).

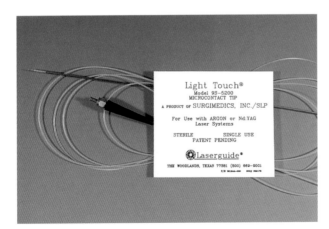

Figure 1.197 A drawn contact tip allows application of the Nd:YAG laser energy to the tissue directly.

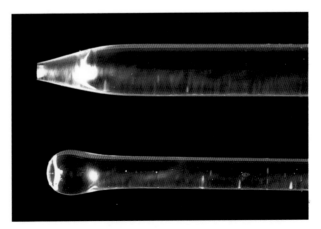

Figure 1.198 The tips are supplied in cone-tip and rounded configurations.

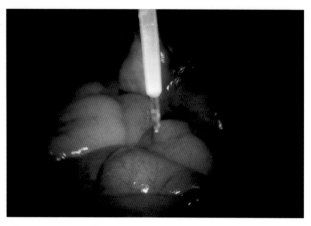

Figure 1.199 The conical tip is used primarily for endoscopic surgery.

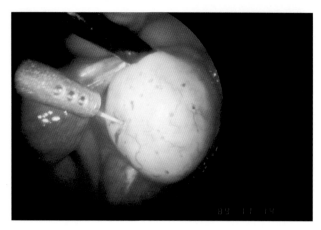

Figure 1.200 The application of the YAG laser with decompression of polycystic ovaries.

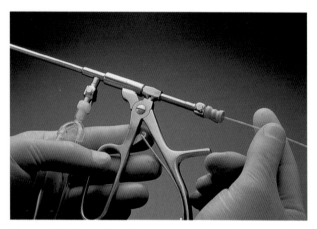

Figure 1.201 A fiber director may be used to aim the fiber through a second-puncture port for appropriate tissue application. A suction-irrigation channel is available (courtesy of Marlow Surgical).

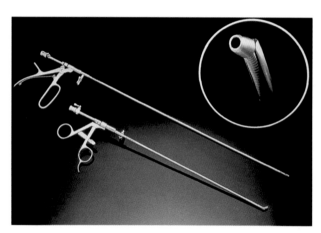

Figure 1.202 A close-up of the fiber director (courtesy of Marlow Surgical).

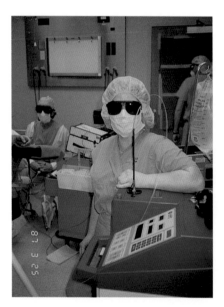

Figure 1.203 Greenish-tinted Nd:YAG laser glasses are needed to protect the retina for the OR personnel and surgeon.

Photodocumentation

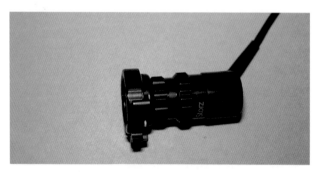

Figure 1.204 The endoscopic CCD chip camera is fastened directly to the end of the endoscope.

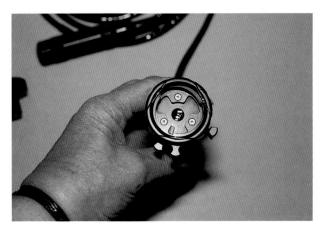

Figure 1.205 The endoscopic CCD chip camera gives the highest resolution when working off the video monitor.

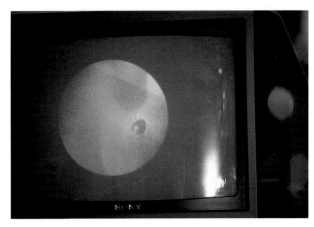

Figure 1.206 A high-resolution video monitor is needed to perform operative laparoscopy or hysteroscopy indirectly.

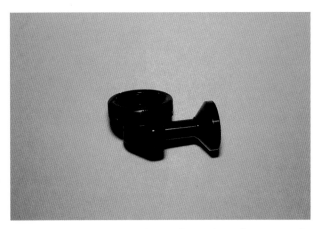

Figure 1.207 A beam splitter allows for videotaping of a procedure while the surgeon views the pelvic pathology directly.

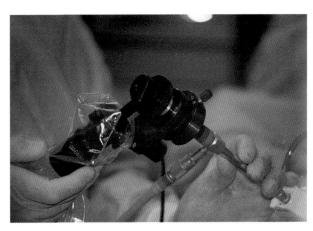

Figure 1.208 The beam splitter is shown attached to the camera and the endoscope.

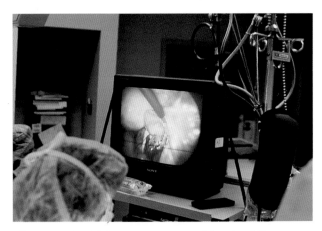

Figure 1.209 This arrangement enables the OR personnel to watch and also allows for documentation for the patient.

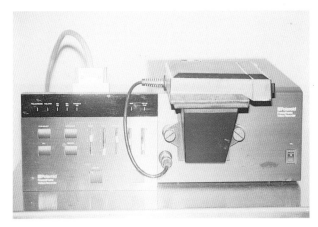

Figure 1.210 A Polaprinter allows for photographing the video image. The pictures are helpful for patient education.

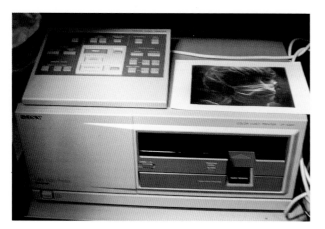

Figure 1.211 A mavigraph takes its picture directly off the electronic signal from the endoscopic camera and gives the best quality for an immediate hard copy.

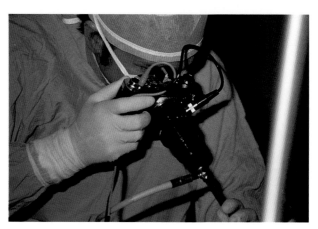

Figure 1.212 35 mm Photodocumentation is needed for slide presentations and/or publication.

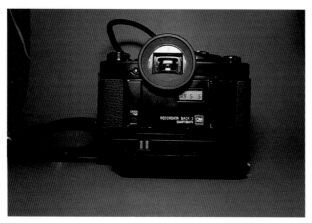

Figure 1.213 35 mm Photodocumentation may be accomplished with an OM-2 camera with motor drive.

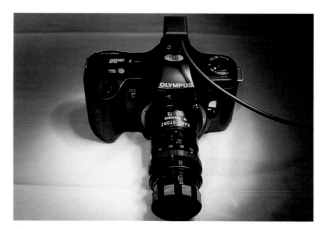

Figure 1.214 35 mm Photodocumentation using an OM-88 camera with a zoom lens attachment.

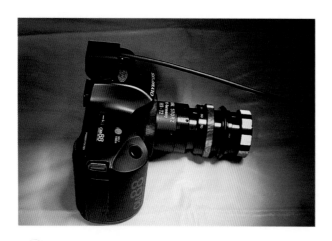

Figure 1.215 A multitude of different image sizes may be obtained through the laparoscope.

Operating room set-up

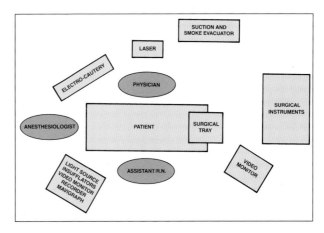

Figure 1.216   Schematic diagram of equipment placement in the OR.

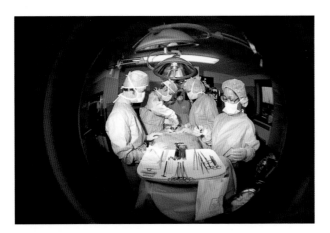

Figure 1.217   The knowledgeable operating team is vital to reduce frustration when performing pelviscopy and operative hysteroscopy. With all the equipment in place, the room may appear quite small.

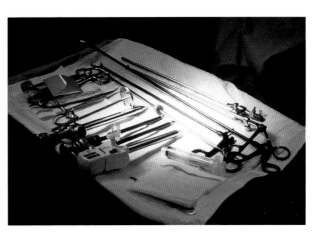

Figure 1.218   The Mayo stand should have all the appropriate instruments immediately accessible for use.

Operating room team

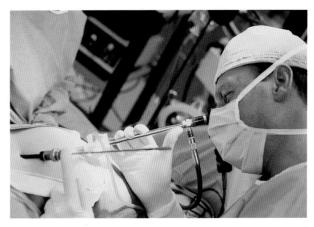

Figure 1.219   The laparoscopist should be able to concentrate on the work at hand by pre-organizing his or her instruments.

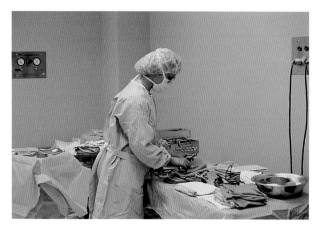

Figure 1.220   The scrub nurse should be well versed on the type of instruments needed and assure their good working order.

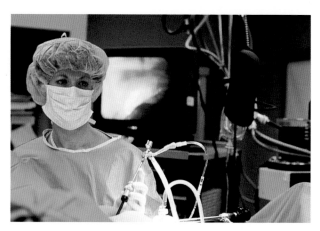

Figure 1.221   An experienced assistant is vital to facilitate difficult operative endoscopic procedures.

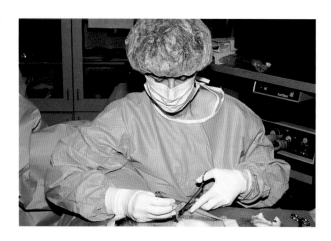

Figure 1.222   A private scrub nurse is helpful in completing wound closure by suturing the skin.

BIBLIOGRAPHY

Azziz R: Operative endoscopy: the pressing need for a structured training and credentialing process. *Fertil Steril* **58**:1100–102, 1992.

Diamond MP (ed): Pelviscopy. In: *Clinical Obstetrics and Gynecology*. Philadelphia, J.B. Lippincott, Vol. 34, p 2, 1991.

Keye W: Hitting a moving target: credentialing the endoscopic surgeon. *Fertil Steril* **62**:1115–19, 1994.

McLaughlin DS (ed): *Lasers in Gynecology*. Philadelphia, J.B. Lippincott, p 81, 1991.

Morales AJ, Murphy AA: Operative laparoscopy in gynecology. In McLucas B, Morales AJ, Murphy AA (eds): *Current Problems in Obstetrics, Gynecology and Fertility*. St. Louis, Mosby Year Book, Vol. 15, 1992.

Reich H: Laparoscopic suturing. *Obstet Gynecol* **79**: 145–54, 1992.

Semm K, Friedrich ER (eds): *Operative Manual for Endoscopic Abdominal Surgery*. Chicago, Yearbook Medical Publishers, 1987.

2 Diagnosis of disease states

Diagnostic laparoscopy and hysteroscopy are invaluable to detect and/or confirm diseases in symptomatic females (Figs 2.1–2.4 and 2.15–2.22). CO_2 is usually the distending medium for each modality, with the flow limited to seven liters per minute electronically in laparoscopy, and 100 ml per minute in hysteroscopy. It is vital to inspect the peritoneal and uterine cavities in a systematic approach in order to avoid overlooking subtle pathologic states, such as endometriosis (Figs 2.5–2.68), adhesions (Figs 2.69–2.125), fibroids (2.126–2.144), developmental anomalies (Figs 2.145–2.164), ovarian disease (Figs 2.165–2.197), ectopic pregnancy (Figs 2.198–2.214), endometrial abnormalities (Figs 2.222–2.242), intra-uterine adhesions (Figs 2.243–2.250), septate uterus (Figs 2.251–2.255), endometrial carcinoma (Figs 2.256–2.259), and miscellaneous uterine diseases (Figs 2.260–2.271). Complete evaluation depends on the gynecological surgeon's knowledge and ability to recognize abnormal states. It is important to consider biopsy if the diagnosis is in question as pathologic confirmation of suspected malignancy is imperative for early diagnosis. The following photographs should help the gynecological endoscopist to recognize common disease states.

Diagnostic laparoscopy

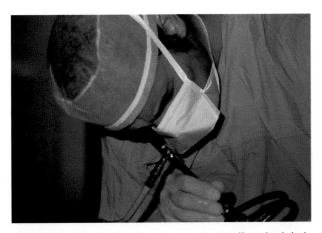

Figure 2.1 Diagnostic laparoscopy is usually scheduled as an outpatient using a 10 mm diagnostic laparoscope inserted through an infra-umbilical incision. The second puncture is placed suprapubicly to manipulate the pelvic organs.

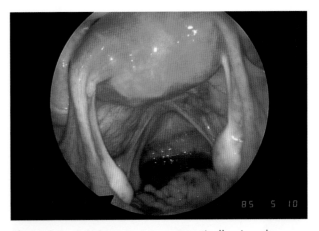

Figure 2.2 It is important to systematically view the pelvic anatomy each time. (a) A general overview of the pelvic organs noting obvious adhesions, a large ovarian cyst, etc. (b) Viewing the right tube and ovary. (c) Viewing the left tube and ovary. (d) Viewing the posterior cul-de-sac. (e) Viewing the anterior cul-de-sac. (f) Checking the bowel, appendix, and upper abdomen as needed.

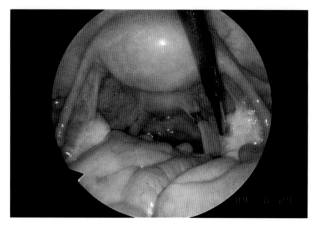

Figure 2.3 In the general overview of Fig. 2.2(a) there appears to be a nodule of endometriosis on the right uterosacral ligament.

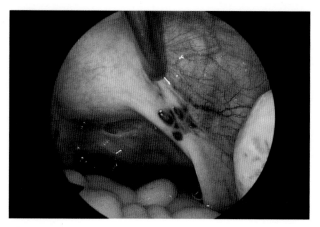

Figure 2.4 Placing the laparoscope closer to pathology magnifies the view and further delineates the pathology.

Endometriosis

Stage I (peritoneal)

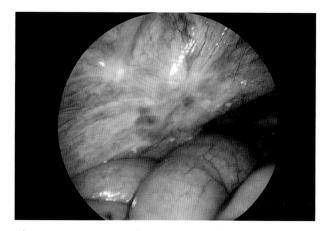

Figure 2.5 Stage I endometriosis, with implants deep to the peritoneal surface.

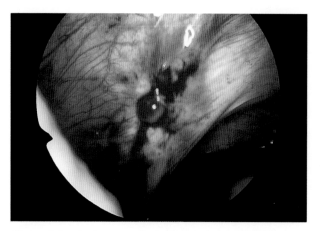

Figure 2.6 Active saccular endometriosis which is bleeding.

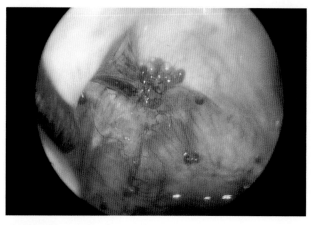

Figure 2.7 Vesicular implants of endometriosis which are exophytic and superficially implanted on the peritoneal surface.

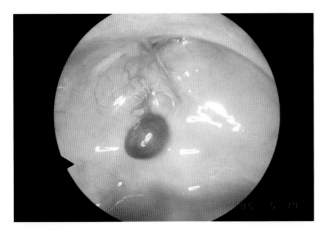

Figure 2.8 Cystic endometriosis on the surface of the peritoneum which resembles a 'blood blister.'

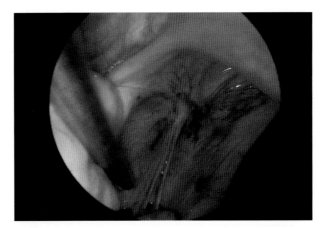

Figure 2.9 Active endometriosis with initial scarring showing contraction of the peritoneal surface and fibrosis.

Allen–Masters Syndrome

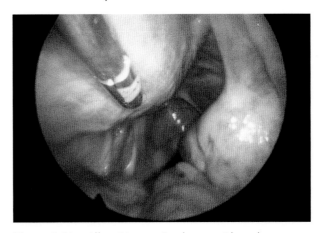

Figure 2.10 A large area of fibrosis with peritoneal contraction secondary to old endometriosis.

Figure 2.11 Allen–Masters Syndrome with early pseudo-sac formation inferior to the right ovary.

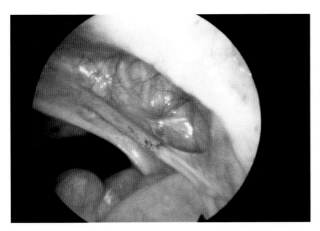

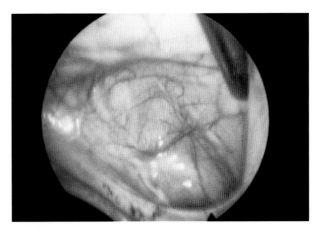

Figure 2.12 Closer view of the internal hernia formed by Allen–Masters Syndrome in this patient.

Figure 2.13 Further close-up view of the internal hernia which often has peritoneal implants of microscopic endometriosis.

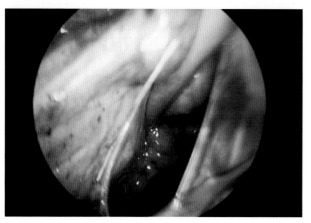

Figure 2.14 The Allen–Masters Syndrome hernia may trap an ovary or a tube and ovary, thus causing pain.

Stage II-A (superficial ovarian)

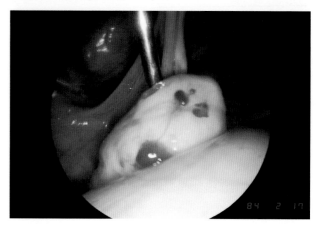

Figure 2.15 Endometriosis stage II-A showing exophytic active implant of ovarian endometriosis.

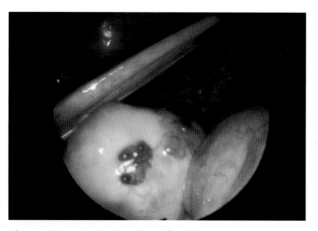

Figure 2.16 Active implant of endometriosis as some begin to penetrate through the ovarian cortex.

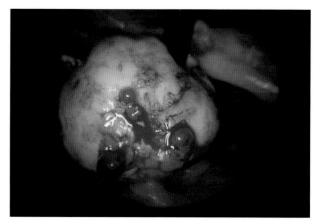

Figure 2.17 Aggressive exophytic hemorrhagic implants of endometriosis on the surface of the ovary.

Stage II-B (deep ovarian)

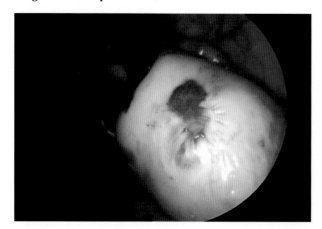

Figure 2.18 Exophytic endometriosis which has penetrated through the ovarian cortex and begun to form a small endometrioma.

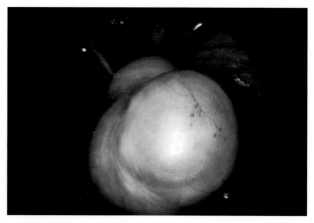

Figure 2.19 An ovarian endometrioma primarily involving the medullary portion of the ovary with minimal signs of surface endometriosis.

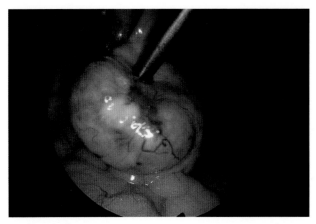

Figure 2.20 Deep and superficial implants of endometriosis showing an early ovarian endometrioma.

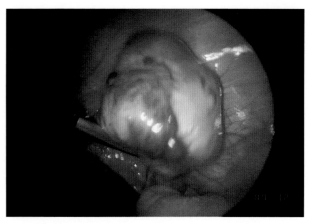

Figure 2.21 Deep endometrioma with multiple loculated areas of old blood forming a chocolate cyst.

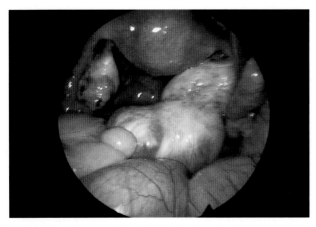

Figure 2.22 Multiple lobes of a loculated endometrioma.

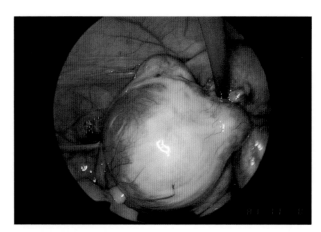

Figure 2.23 Deep endometrioma encompassing 90% of the ovary.

Ovarian adhesions

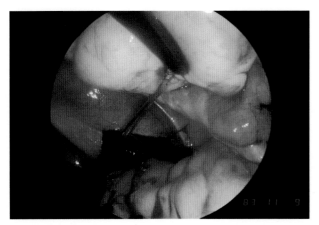

Figure 2.24 Early adhesion formation between the ovary containing an endometrioma (endometriosis stage II-B).

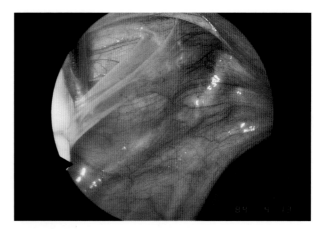

Figure 2.25 Early filmy adhesions from an endometriosis-associated endometrioma.

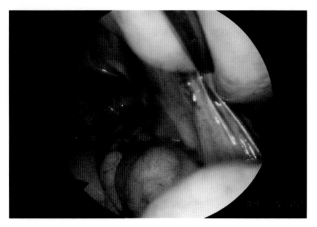

Figure 2.26 Fibrotic dense adhesion formation from ovarian endometrioma.

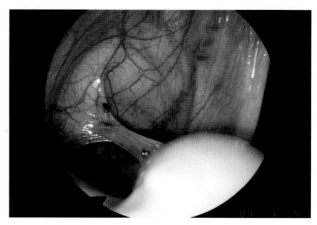

Figure 2.27 Active implants of endometriosis seen on the adhesion binding the left ovary to the left lateral pelvic wall.

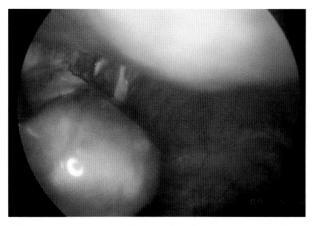

Figure 2.28 Dense adhesions binding the ovary to the posterior surface of the left lateral pelvic wall and uterus.

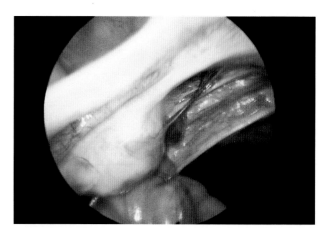

Figure 2.29 Banjo string and dense adhesions binding the ovary to the left lateral pelvic wall.

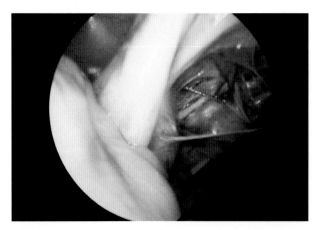

Figure 2.30 Banjo string adhesions with an ovarian endometrioma attaching it to the left lateral pelvic wall.

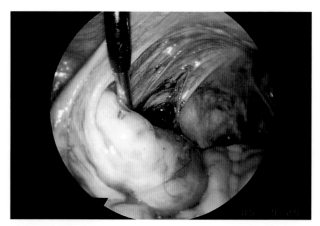

Figure 2.31 A deep endometrioma, entered as the probe attempted to mobilize the ovary by bluntly lysing the adhesions binding the ovary to the left lateral pelvic wall.

Ruptured endometriomas

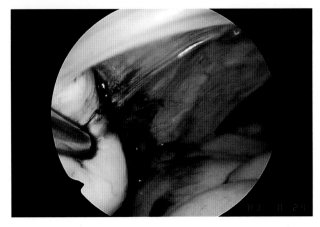

Figure 2.32 Deep endometrioma beginning to exude a 'Hershey syrup-type' exudate as the left ovary is attempted to be mobilized.

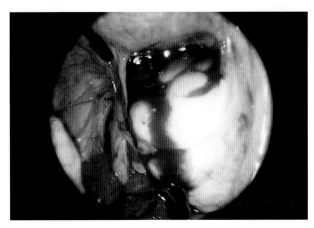

Figure 2.33 Ruptured endometrioma with deep endometrial glands producing a chocolate cyst and dense adhesions binding the right ovary to the posterior uterus and right lateral pelvic wall.

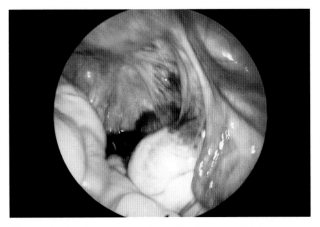

Figure 2.34 Dense adhesions binding the right ovary with a ruptured endometrioma to the ureter and sidewall.

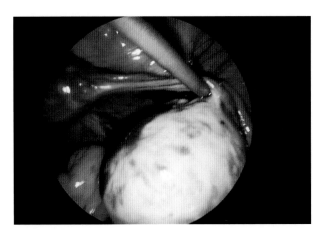

Figure 2.35 7.5 cm right endometrioma initially ruptured upon attempted blunt mobilization.

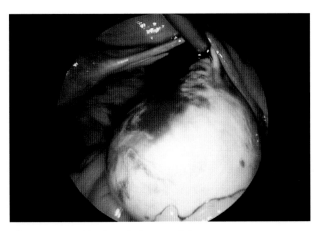

Figure 2.36 Further drainage of the same endometrioma following further manipulation.

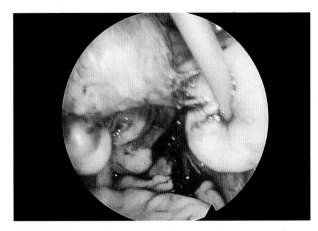

Figure 2.37 Another endometrioma which ruptured upon blunt mobilization of the right ovary.

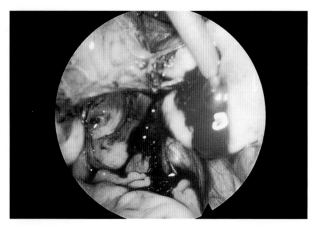

Figure 2.38 Close-up of the endometrioma as it continues to drain.

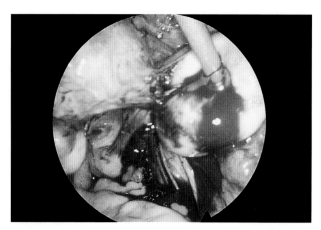

Figure 2.39 Irrigation of the endometrioma by the suction-irrigation probe, as the chocolate-like fluid exudes from the ovarian defect.

Stage III (tubal)

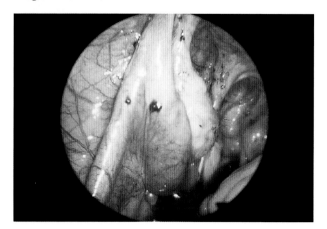

Figure 2.40 Further drainage and irrigation of the same endometrioma.

Figure 2.41 Stage III endometriosis showing serosal implants of endometriosis on the fallopian tube.

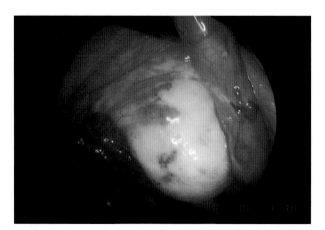

Figure 2.42 Tubal endometriosis (stage III) with peritoneal constricture and some narrowing of the right tube.

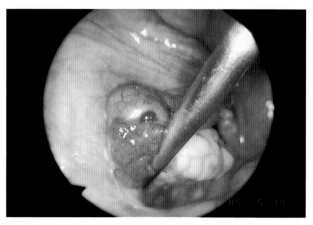

Figure 2.43 Distal tubal endometriosis just proximal to the left fimbria.

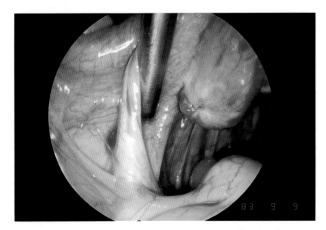

Figure 2.44 Fimbrial endometriosis with distal tubal occlusion secondary to pelvic inflammatory disease.

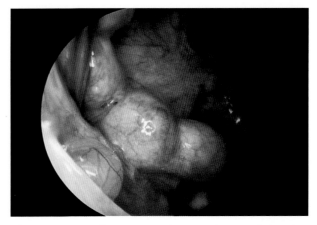

Figure 2.45 Mid-segment endometriosis constricting the left fallopian tube.

Stage IV (GI/GU)

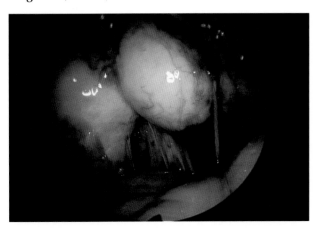

Figure 2.46 Endometriosis stage IV with bilaterally large endometriomas and severe pelvic adhesions in the posterior cul-de-sac ('kissing ovaries').

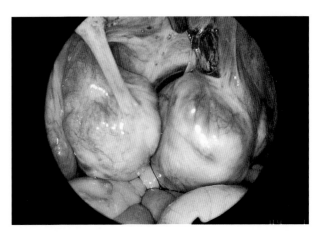

Figure 2.47 Bilateral large endometriomas adherent to the posterior cul-de-sac lateral pelvic wall.

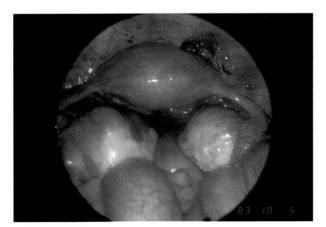

Figure 2.48 Stage IV disease with bilateral large endometriomas obliterating the posterior cul-de-sac with right bladder implant.

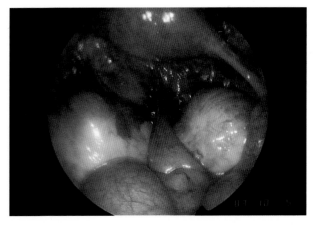

Figure 2.49 Closer view of the patient of Fig. 2.48 shows the dense adhesions and endometriotic fluid in the cul-de-sac.

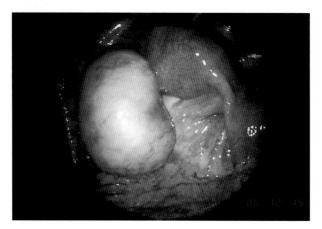

Figure 2.50   Endometriosis stage IV showing a predominantly enlarged left ovary containing a deep endometrioma.

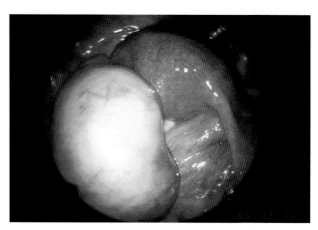

Figure 2.51   Closer view of the endometrioma.

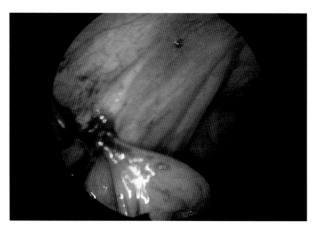

Figure 2.52   Endometriosis stage IV involving the left ureter with an endometrial adhesive bridge attaching the epiploic fat of the bowel to the left lateral pelvic sidewall.

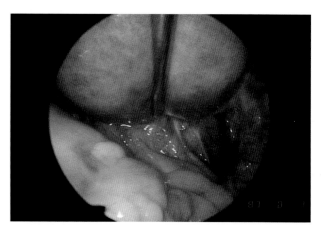

Figure 2.53   Dense adhesions in the posterior cul-de-sac between the bowel and posterior vagina due to extensive endometriosis.

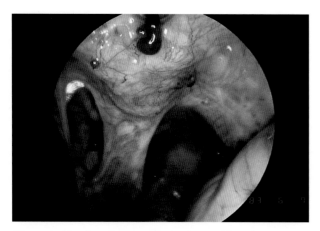

Figure 2.54   Exophytic endometriosis with a dense fibrotic bridge to the rectum.

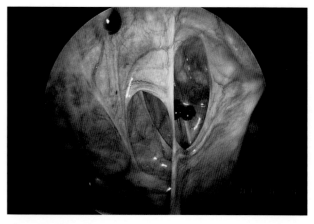

Figure 2.55   Closer view of the very dense adhesions with saccular endometriosis.

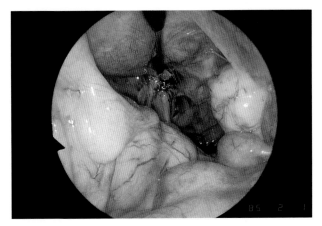

Figure 2.56 Dense aggressive adhesions between the uterus, posterior vagina, and large bowel.

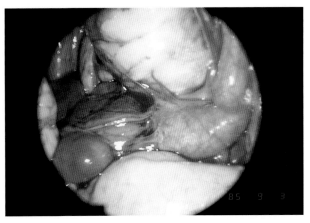

Figure 2.57 Obliterated cul-de-sac with involvement of the ovary, ureter, right tube, and large bowel.

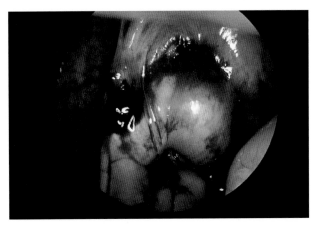

Figure 2.58 Dense adhesions attaching the rectum to the posterior vagina due to nodular endometriosis.

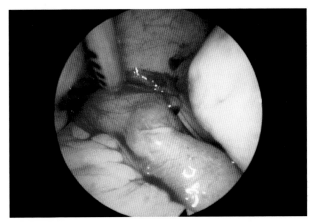

Figure 2.59 Bowel implants of endometriosis attaching the rectum to the posterior vagina.

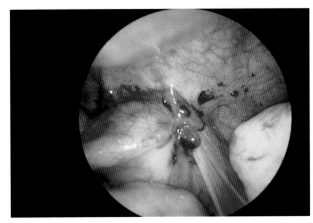

Figure 2.60 Tenting of the bowel with fibrotic attachment of the large bowel to the posterior vagina. This lesion extended more than half-way through the bowel wall and required bowel resection at laparotomy.

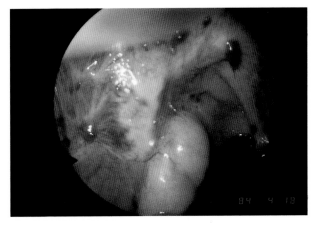

Figure 2.61 Deep bowel endometriosis with aggressive sub-serosal and exophytic lesions attaching the bowel to the posterior vagina.

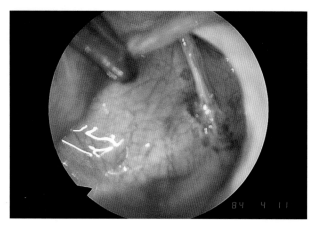

Figure 2.62 Serosal and partial thickness penetration of the large bowel by endometrial implants.

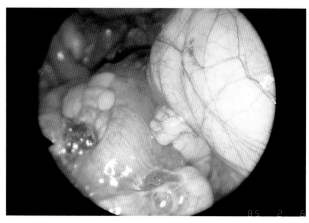

Figure 2.63 Exophytic implants of endometriosis on the large bowel serosa.

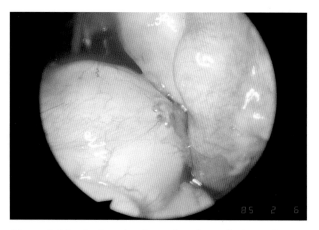

Figure 2.64 Surface implant of endometriosis on the small bowel.

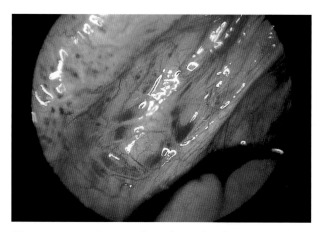

Figure 2.65 Left ureteral implant of endometriosis.

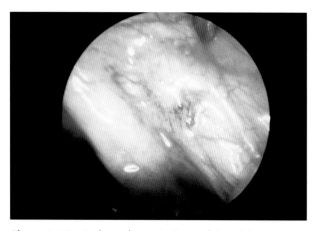

Figure 2.66 Early endometriosis overlying right ureter.

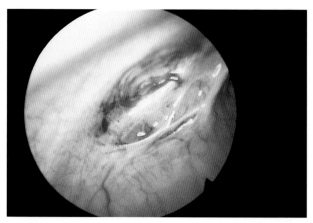

Figure 2.67 Left ureteral involvement of endometriosis with early fibrosis.

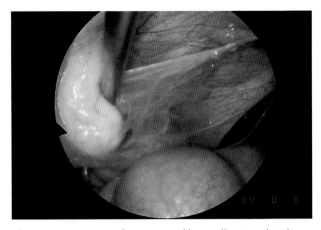

Figure 2.79 Post-inflammatory filmy adhesions binding the left ovary to the left lateral pelvic wall.

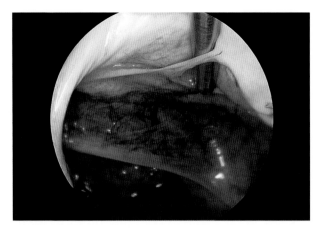

Figure 2.80 Dense adhesion binding the left ovary to the left posterior uterus and left lateral pelvic wall.

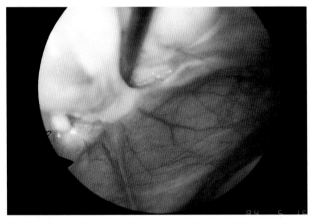

Figure 2.81 Dense adhesions binding the left ovary to the left lateral pelvic wall.

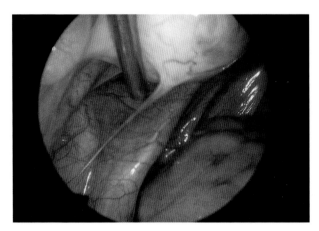

Figure 2.82 Banjo string adhesion binding the left ovary to the left lateral pelvic wall.

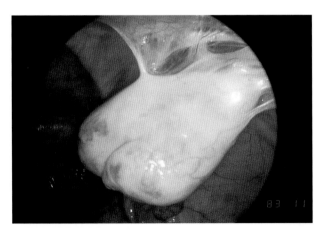

Figure 2.83 Dense adhesions binding the right ovary to the anterior abdominal wall due to previous surgery with post-operative infection.

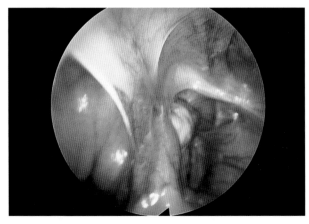

Figure 2.84 Dense adhesions involving the right adnexa and the anterior abdominal wall.

Bowel

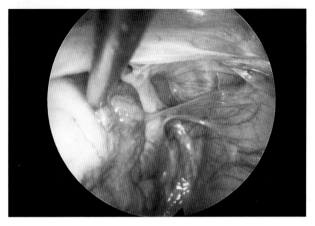

Figure 2.85 Dense adhesions involving the appendix and ileocecal valve to the abdominal wall.

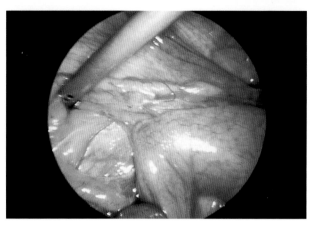

Figure 2.86 Dense adhesions involving the small bowel to the lateral pelvic wall.

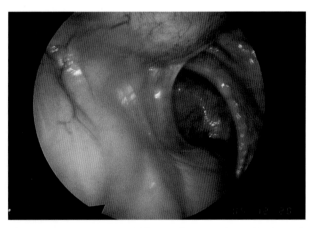

Figure 2.87 Dense and filmy adhesions from the bowel to the uterus overlying the left adnexa.

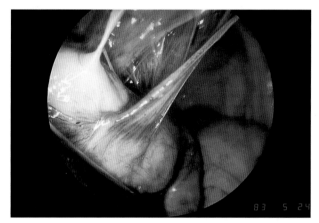

Figure 2.88 Dense adhesions encompassing the left ovary.

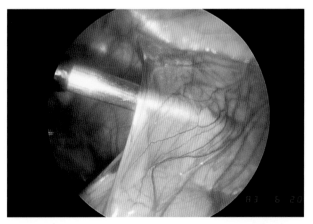

Figure 2.89 Congenital band from the bowel to the right lateral pelvic wall.

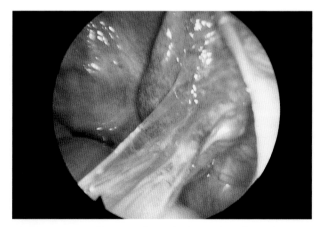

Figure 2.90 Adhesions from the bowel to the right tube.

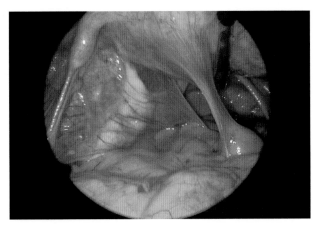

Figure 2.91 Dense adhesions from a loop of small bowel to the posterior fundus of the uterus with filmy adhesions attaching the bowel to the left adnexa and posterior uterus. This patient had symptoms of intermittent small bowel obstruction.

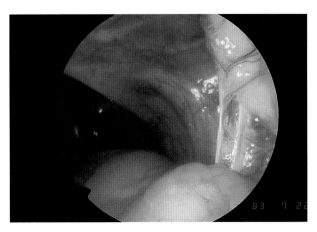

Figure 2.92 Adhesions of large bowel to right adnexa.

Tubal

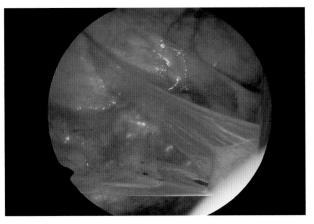

Figure 2.93 Filmy adhesions from the bowel to the left lateral anterior abdominal wall.

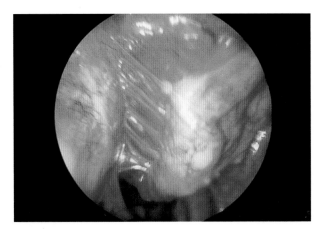

Figure 2.94 Filmy adhesions from the left tube to the left lateral pelvic wall, restricting tubal motility. Note healthy fimbria.

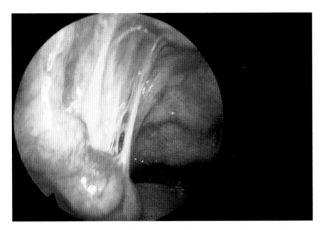

Figure 2.95 Filmy adhesions and dense adhesions from the left tube to the posterior uterus and lateral wall.

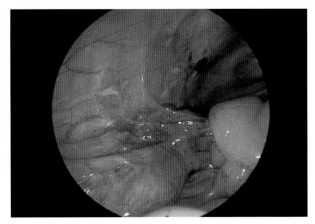

Figure 2.96 Epiploic fat adherent to the left lateral pelvic wall and the remaining left tube and ovary (Residual Ovary Syndrome).

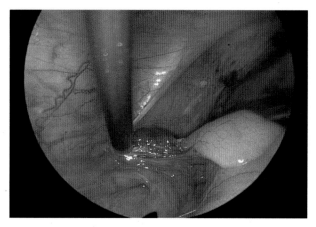

Figure 2.97 Close-up view of the same patient. Note how the ovary is encompassed by the dense adhesions.

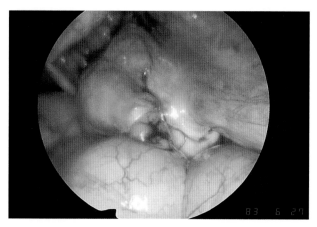

Figure 2.98 Distal serosal narrowing has not appreciably damaged the healthy fimbria.

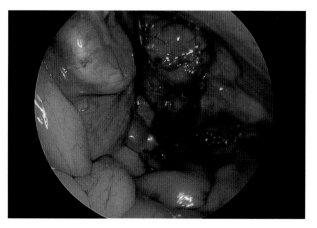

Figure 2.99 Tubal adhesions, but patent tube with healthy fimbria.

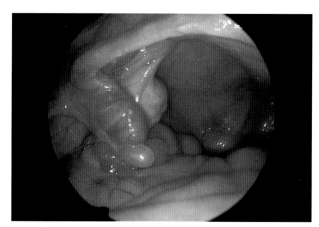

Figure 2.100 Tubal adhesions immobilizing and kinking the left tube. On hysterosalpingogram the tube would appear patent, but is markedly impaired for ovum pick-up.

Tubal phimosis

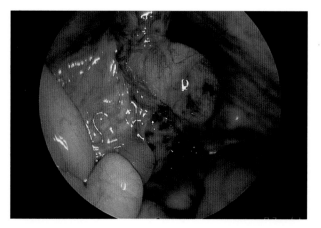

Figure 2.101 Marked tubal phimosis with fairly healthy fimbria.

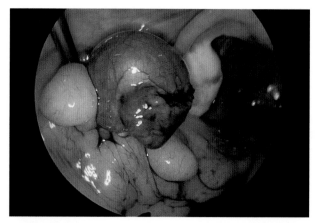

Figure 2.102 Marked tubal phimosis with hydrosalpinx which evolved during hydrotubation of methylene blue dye injected transcervically.

Distal tubal occlusion

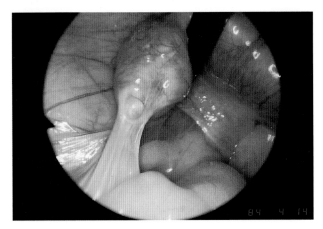

Figure 2.103 True distal tubal occlusion with adhesion from the distal tube to the small bowel. Note the blue dye inside the tube with a dimple at the apex of the fimbrial agglutination.

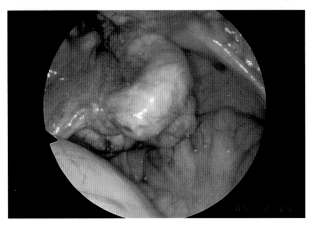

Figure 2.104 Distal tubal occlusion with a mild hydrosalpinx.

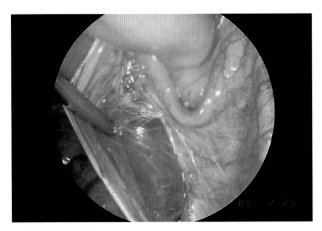

Figure 2.105 Distal tubal occlusion of pelvic adhesions.

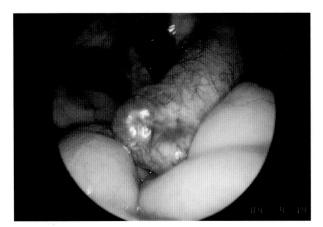

Figure 2.106 Marked distal inflammatory tubal occlusion.

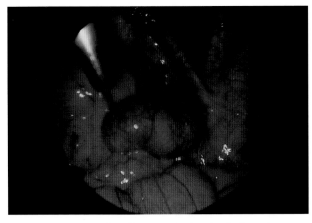

Figure 2.107 Hydrosalpinx with distal tubal occlusion.

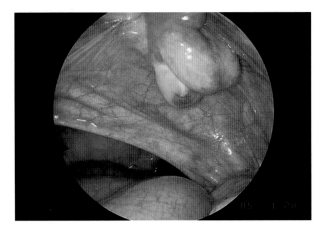

Figure 2.108 Distal tubal occlusion, post-inflammatory with a mild hydrosalpinx.

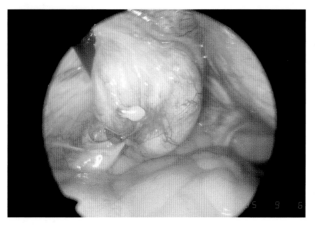

Figure 2.109 Distal tubal occlusion. Again note the agglutinated apex of the fimbria.

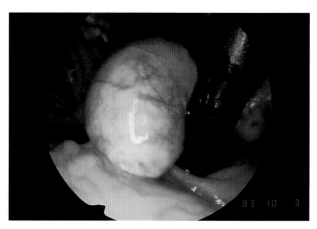

Figure 2.110 Hydrosalpinx with distal tubal occlusion.

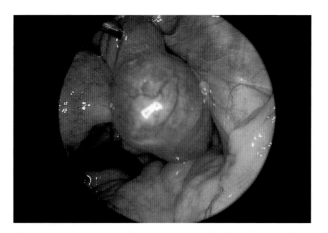

Figure 2.111 Larger hydrosalpinx, which is thin-walled.

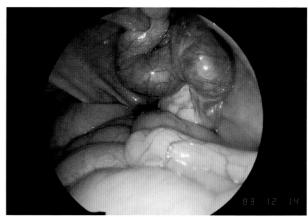

Figure 2.112 Tortuous hydrosalpinx showing the tint of blue dye.

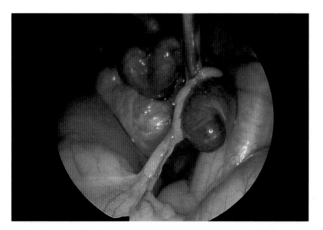

Figure 2.113 Markedly tortuous hydrosalpinx with distal tubal occlusion, filled with blue dye.

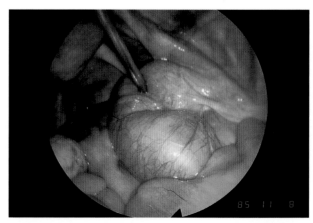

Figure 2.114 Saccular tubal hydrosalpinx with distal tubal occlusion.

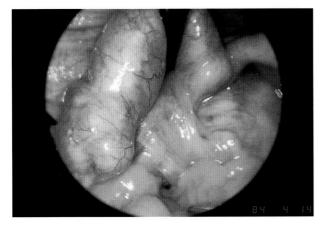

Figure 2.115 Hydrosalpinx secondary to tubal occlusion.

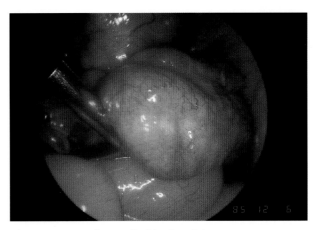

Figure 2.116 Thin-walled hydrosalpinx.

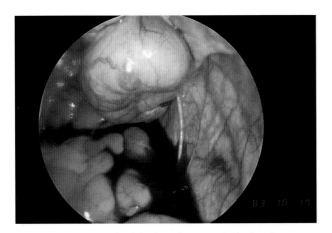

Figure 2.117 Marked hydrosalpinx with fimbrial agglutination.

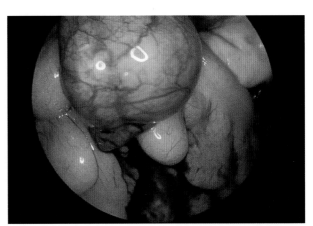

Figure 2.118 Marked hydrosalpinx distended by blue dye.

Mid-segment occlusion

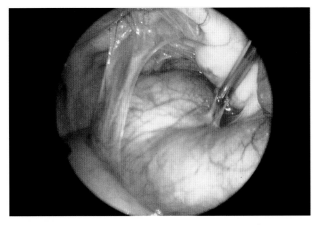

Figure 2.119 Severely damaged tube, hydrosalpinx, and adhesions.

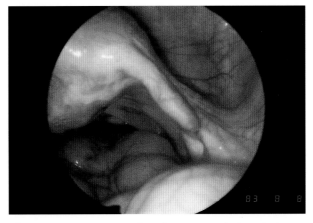

Figure 2.120 Congenital mid-segment tubal occlusion with distal tubal atrophy.

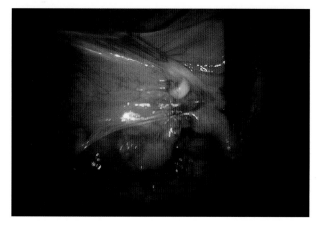

Figure 2.121 Iatrogenic mid-segment tubal occlusion due to Fallope ring.

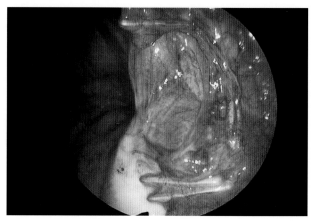

Figure 2.122 Mid-segment tubal occlusion due to tubal clips.

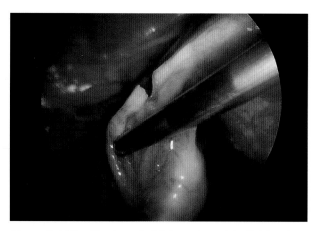

Figure 2.123 Bipolar tubal fulgeration with division by scissors.

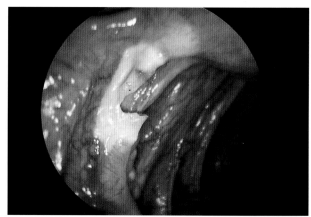

Figure 2.124 Cornual tubal occlusion secondary to bipolar tubal cautery and division.

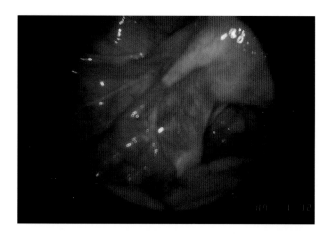

Figure 2.125 Previous mid-segment tubal excision following post-partum ligation.

Fibroids

Subserosal

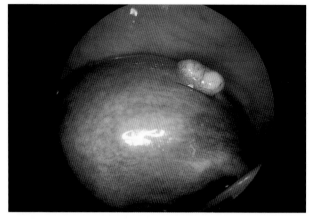

Figure 2.126 Small subserosal fibroids on anterior uterine wall.

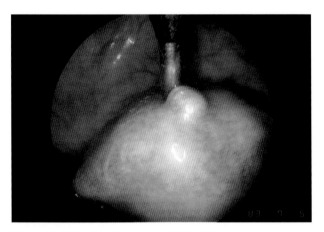

Figure 2.127 Small subserosal fibroid.

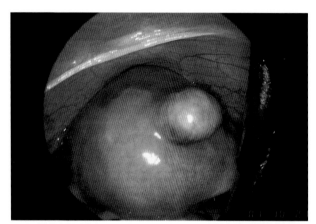

Figure 2.128 Intramural and larger subserosal fibroid.

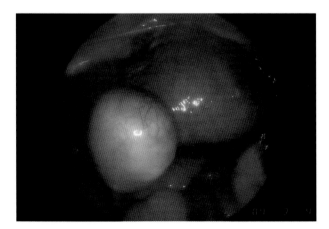

Figure 2.129 Left cornual fibroid.

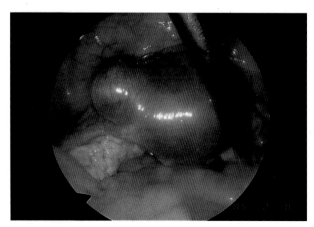

Figure 2.130 Cornual fibroid.

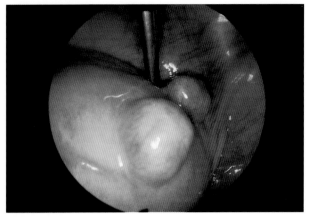

Figure 2.131 Multiple subserosal fibroids.

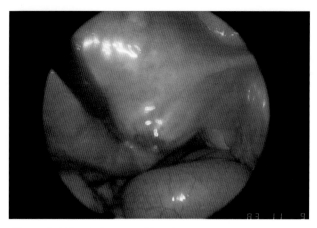

Figure 2.132 Adenomyofibrosis.

Interligamentous

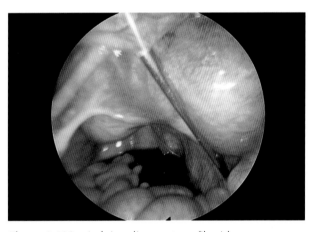

Figure 2.133 Left interligamentous fibroid.

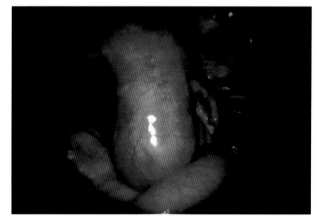

Figure 2.134 Large intramural posterior fibroid.

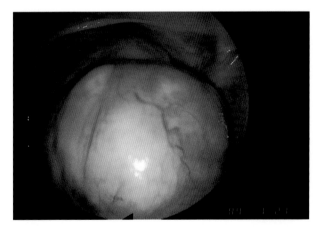

Figure 2.135 Degenerating fibroid which has become calcified.

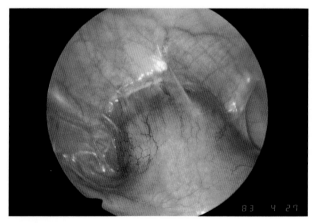

Figure 2.136 Anterior fundal fibroid with adhesion formation.

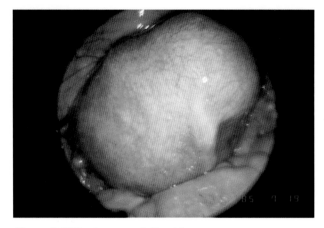

Figure 2.137   Intramural fibroid.

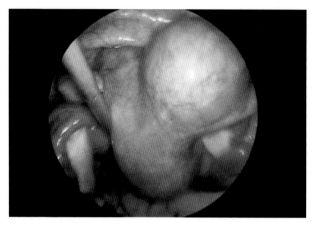

Figure 2.138   Multiple intramural subserosal fibroids.

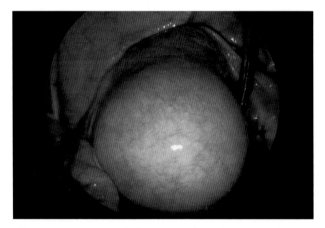

Figure 2.139   Large left posterior-lateral intramural fibroid.

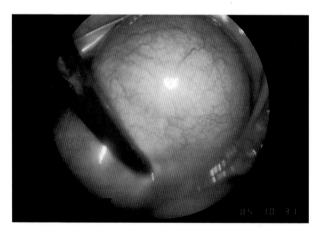

Figure 2.140   Right intramural fibroid arising medial to the insertion of the round ligament.

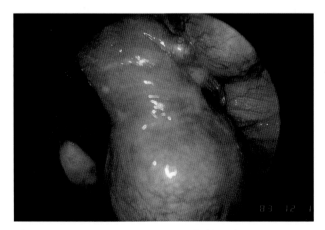

Figure 2.141   Larger posterior wall fibroid.

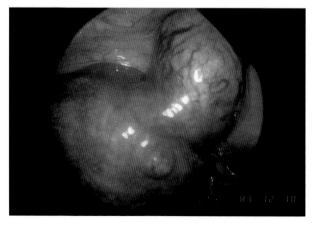

Figure 2.142   Same patient of Fig. 2.141 with right cornual fibroid.

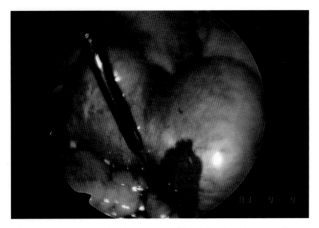

Figure 2.143 Multiple uterine fibroids showing uterine perforation from uterine sound.

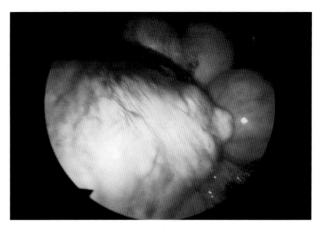

Figure 2.144 Multiple uterine fibroids.

Developmental anomalies

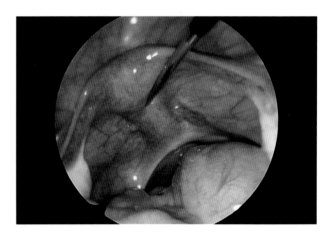

Figure 2.145 Diethylstilbestrol-(DES)-exposed T-shaped uterus.

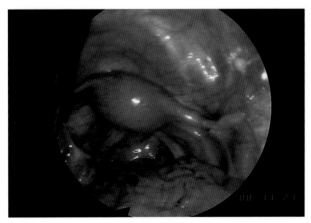

Figure 2.146 DES-exposed uterus.

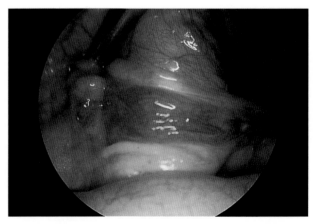

Figure 2.147 Turner Syndrome with uterine hypoplasia.

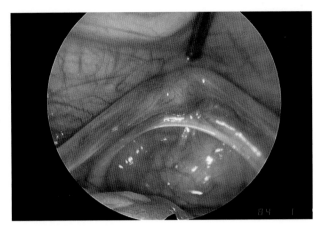

Figure 2.148   Turner Syndrome with uterine hypoplasia.

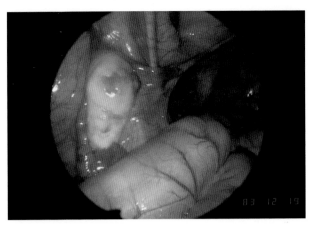

Figure 2.149   Congenital absence of left proximal fallopian tube.

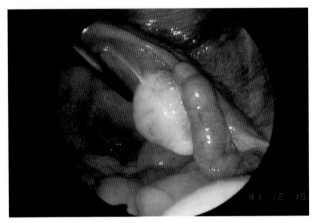

Figure 2.150   Congenital absence of right proximal fallopian tube.

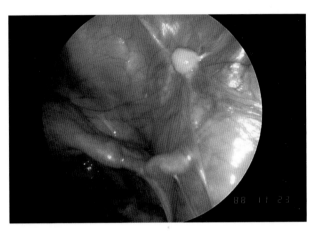

Figure 2.151   Hypoplasia right ovary.

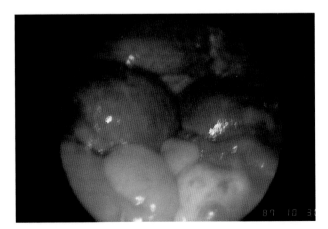

Figure 2.152   True bicornuate uterus.

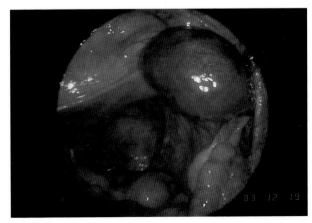

Figure 2.153   Right unicornuate uterus.

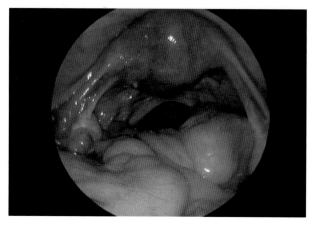

Figure 2.154 Septate uterus—note slightly widened fundus with thickened mid-segment.

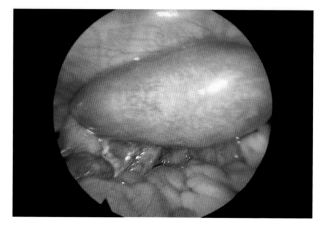

Figure 2.155 Septate uterus with wide fundus and slightly larger right horn.

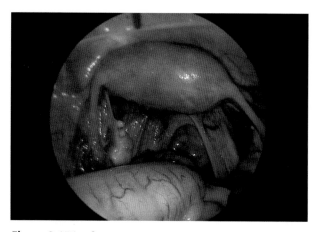

Figure 2.156 Septate uterus.

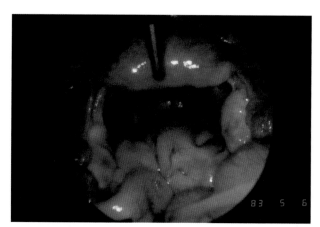

Figure 2.157 Septate uterus.

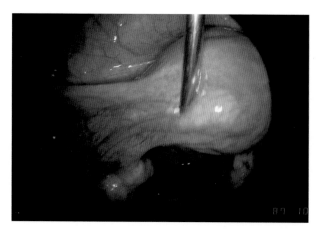

Figure 2.158 Left cornual polyp—note swelling at the insertion of the left fallopian tube.

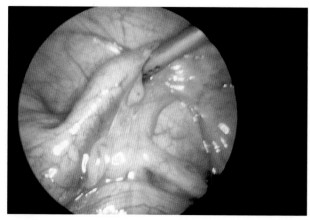

Figure 2.159 Meckel's diverticulum.

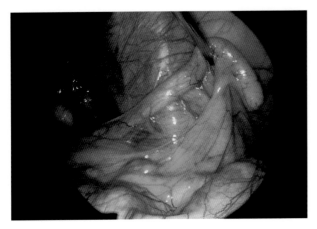

Figure 2.160   Normal appendix.

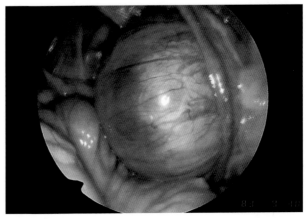

Figure 2.161   Paraovarian cyst distorting the right tubal anatomy.

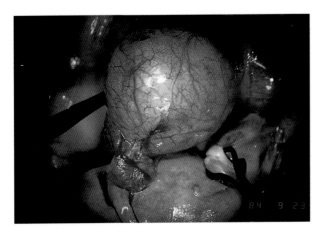

Figure 2.162   Distal left paraovarian cyst.

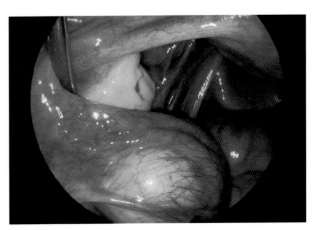

Figure 2.163   Large left paraovarian cyst.

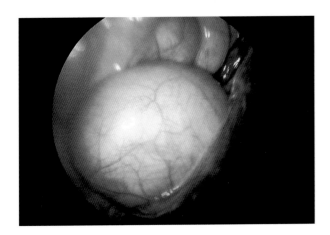

Figure 2.164   Paraovarian cyst.

Ovaries

Polycystic ovaries

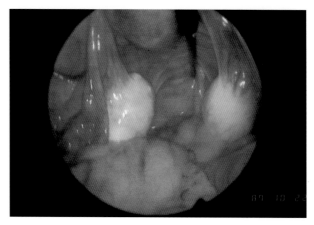

Figure 2.165 Polycystic ovaries. Note the elongated uterovarian ligaments and multiple subcapsular cysts.

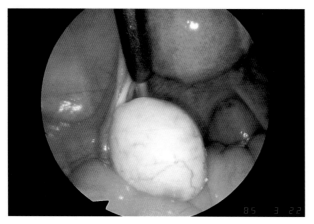

Figure 2.166 Typical polycystic ovaries with marked androgen excess. Note the smooth capsule surface of the enlarged ovary.

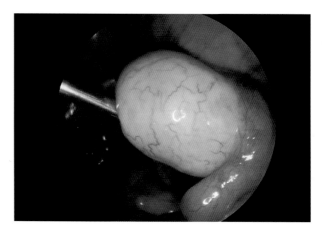

Figure 2.167 Polycystic ovaries.

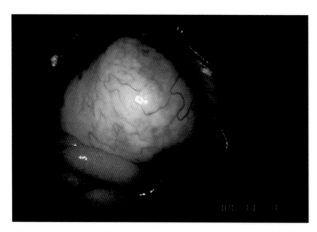

Figure 2.168 Polycystic ovaries.

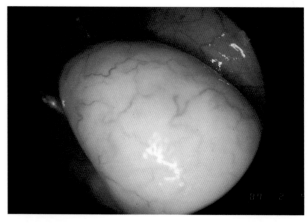

Figure 2.169 Larger polycystic ovary. Patient had severe oligomenorrhea with endometrial hyperplasia.

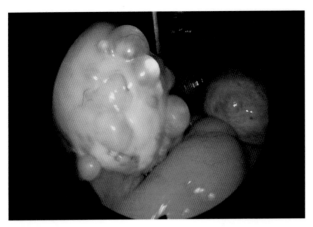

Figure 2.170 Multiple capsular cysts with cortical excrescences. Pathologically polycystic ovaries were confirmed with no malignancy.

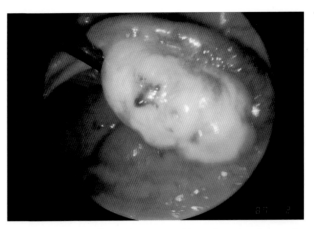

Figure 2.171 Polycystic ovary with surface implants of endometriosis. Oligo-ovulation and endometriosis are often associated.

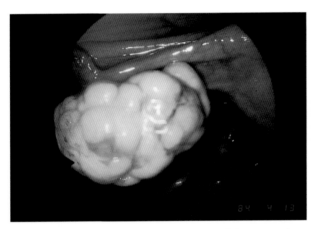

Figure 2.172 Polycystic ovaries with nodular cortical cysts.

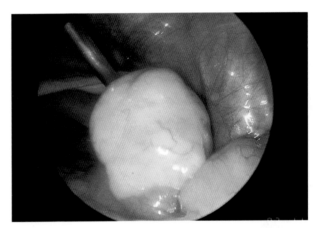

Figure 2.173 Polycystic ovaries—patient on oral contraceptives.

Corpus luteum cysts

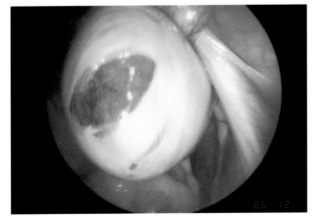

Figure 2.174 Ruptured right corpus luteum cyst following a spontaneous ovulation.

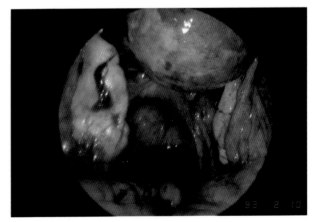

Figure 2.175 Hemorrhagic corpus luteum cyst in a patient with a rare coagulopathy.

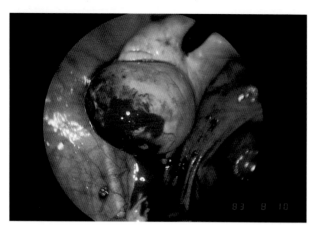

Figure 2.176 Close-up of the actively hemorrhaging corpus luteum cyst.

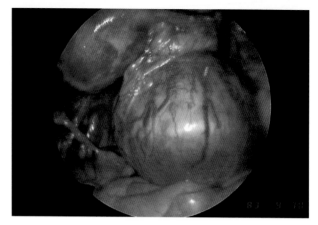

Figure 2.177 Serous cystadenoma.

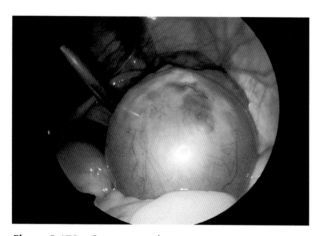

Figure 2.178 Serous cystadenoma.

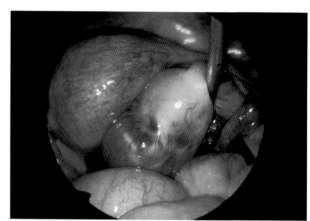

Figure 2.179 Another view of the same patient as in Figs 2.177 and 2.178 with a serous cystadenoma.

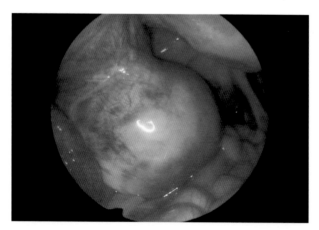

Figure 2.180 Serous cystadenoma.

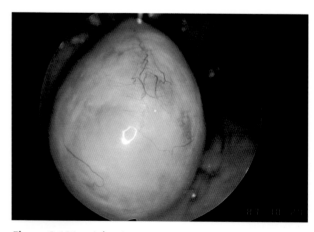

Figure 2.181 A benign serous cyst.

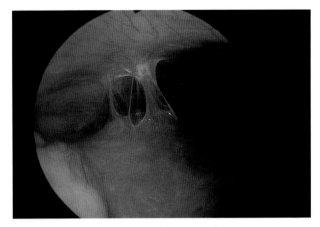

Figure 2.182   A benign serous cyst.

Figure 2.183   Serous cystadenoma with adhesion formation.

Pseudomucinous cysts

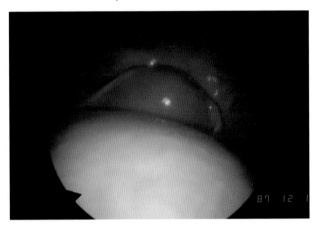

Figure 2.184   Pseudomucinous cystadenoma.

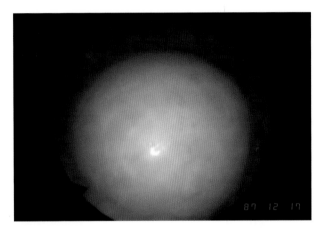

Figure 2.185   Another view of the pseudomucinous cystadenoma of Fig. 2.184.

Solid tumors

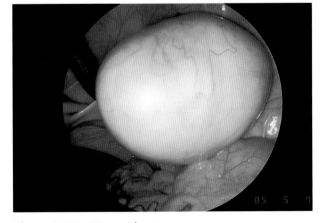

Figure 2.186   Dermoid cyst.

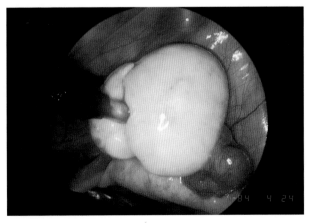

Figure 2.187   Ovarian fibroma-thecoma.

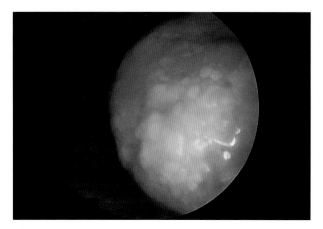

Figure 2.188 Benign serous cystadenoma with multiple cortical excrescences.

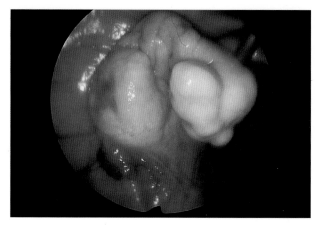

Figure 2.189 Multiple benign loculations.

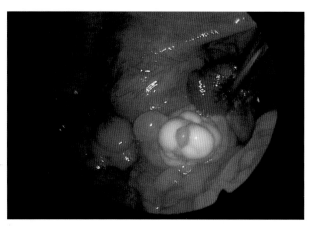

Figure 2.190 Benign serous cystadenomas with a fibroma.

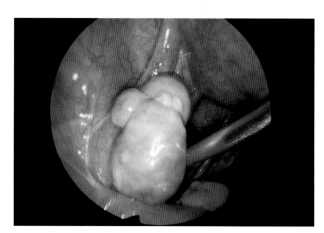

Figure 2.191 Ovarian fibromas.

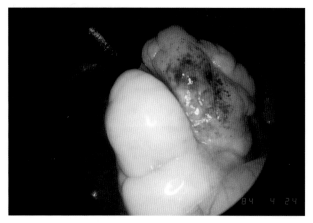

Figure 2.192 Ovarian fibroma-thecoma.

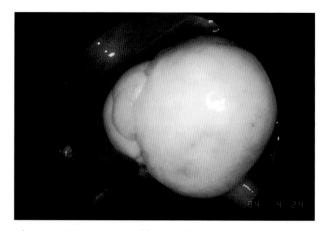

Figure 2.193 Ovarian fibroma-thecoma.

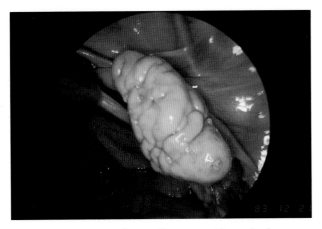

Figure 2.194 Granulosa cell tumor with marked yellowish discoloration.

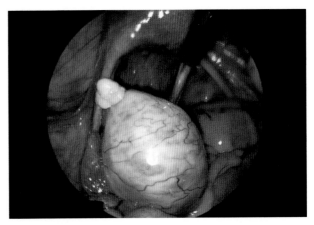

Figure 2.195 Ovarian fibroma.

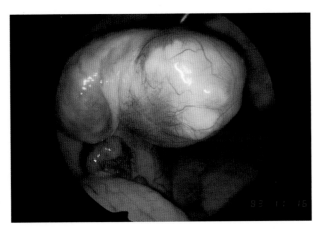

Figure 2.196 Ovarian fibroid.

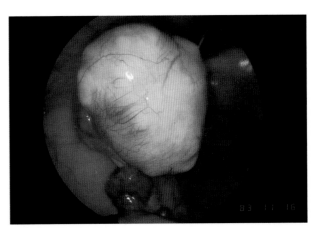

Figure 2.197 Close-up of ovarian fibroid.

Ectopic pregnancy

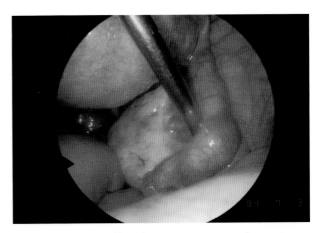

Figure 2.198 Small mid-segment unruptured ectopic. Ectopic pregnancies are unique to humans, occur in 2% of all pregnancies, and a corpus luteum cyst is found in the opposite ovary 25% of the time.

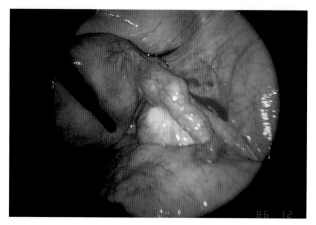

Figure 2.199 Unruptured ectopic pregnancy. A fetus is found in 50% of the ectopic pregnancies.

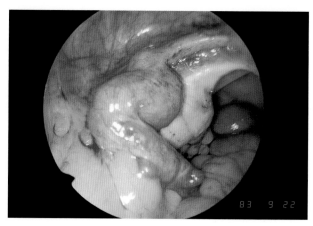

Figure 2.200 Larger unruptured mid-segment ectopic pregnancy. Fewer chromosomal abnormalities are detected in ectopic pregnancies than in spontaneous abortions.

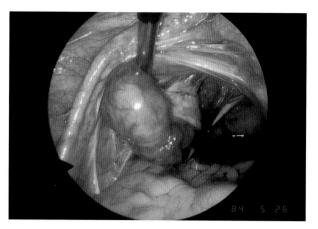

Figure 2.201 Larger ectopic pregnancy. Etiology of ectopics includes sexually transmitted diseases, intra-uterine device (IUD) failures, congenital anomalies (DES exposure, accessory tubal ostia), and infertility treatments (sterilization reversal, reconstructive tubal surgery, ovulation induction, and assisted reproductive technology).

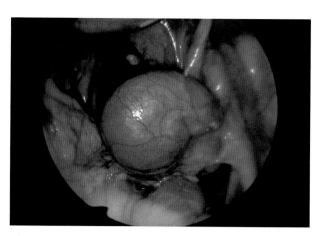

Figure 2.202 Larger right tubal ectopic pregnancy with hemorrhage.

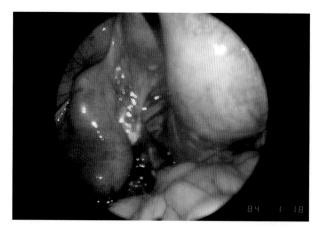

Figure 2.203 Left ectopic pregnancy involving two-thirds of the tube with hemorrhage.

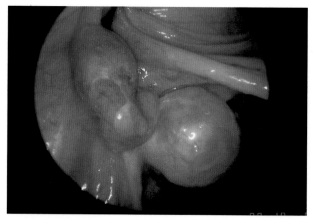

Figure 2.204 Distal left ectopic pregnancy.

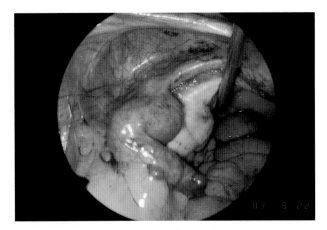

Figure 2.205   Mid-segment left ectopic pregnancy.

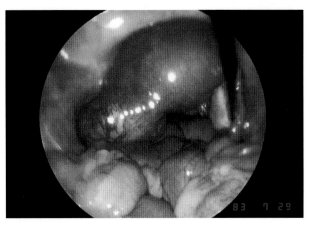

Figure 2.206   Left cornual ectopic pregnancy.

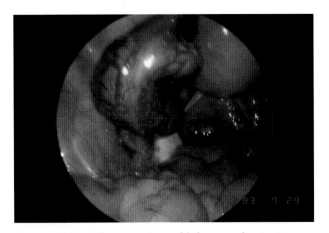

Figure 2.207   Close-up view of left cornual ectopic.

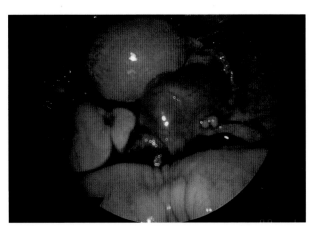

Figure 2.208   Hemorrhagic right ectopic pregnancy with involvement of entire right tube.

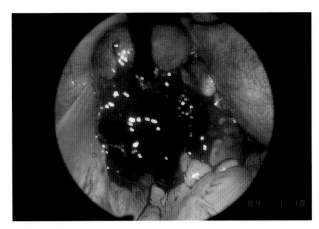

Figure 2.209   Ruptured left ectopic pregnancy with hemorrhage exuding through the fimbria.

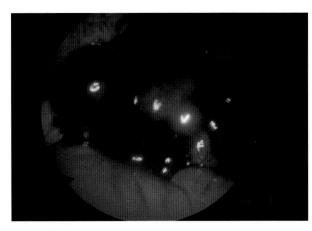

Figure 2.210   Ruptured ectopic pregnancy.

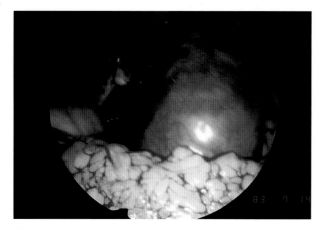

Figure 2.211 Large ruptured ectopic pregnancy.

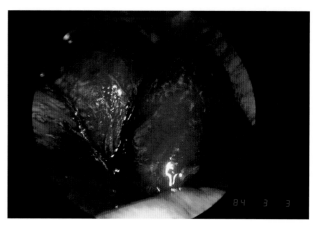

Figure 2.212 Large ruptured ectopic pregnancy with hemoperitoneum.

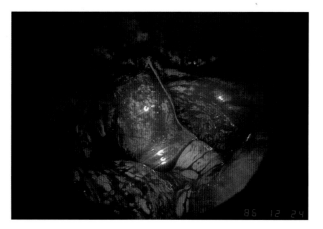

Figure 2.213 Ruptured ectopic pregnancy presented in shock. Usually, either the patient presents as hypotensive or the ectopic is found in asymptomatic infertility patients. Less than 20% rupture in most medical centers.

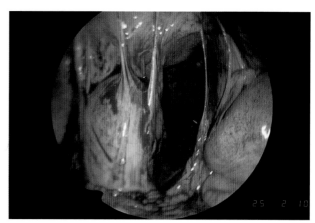

Figure 2.214 Ectopic pregnancy with hemorrhage and bowel adhesions; 90% of patients with ectopic pregnancy have pain, vaginal bleeding, and an adnexal mass.

Diagnostic hysteroscopy

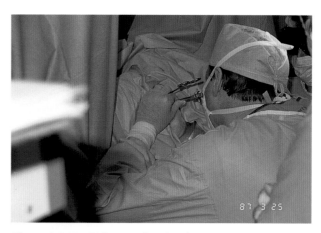

Figure 2.215 When performing hysteroscopy it is important to systematically review the endometrial cavity; first look at the mid-line of the fundus, then each tubal ostia, and finally the lower uterine segment.

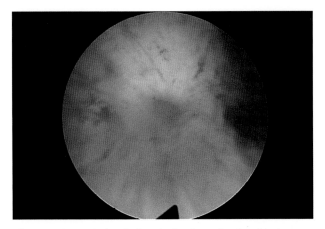

Figure 2.216 Left tubal ostia is viewed using Hyskon as the distending medium.

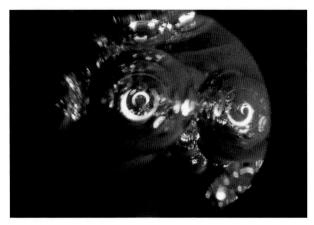

Figure 2.217 Bubbles may be encountered when using Hyskon.

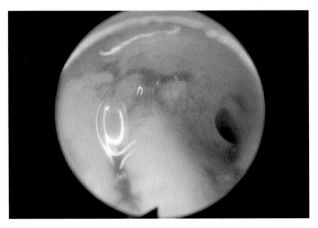

Figure 2.218 Tubal ostia seen using CO_2 as the distending medium.

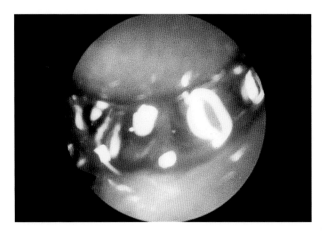

Figure 2.219 Bubbles may also be encountered with CO_2 if moisture is encountered.

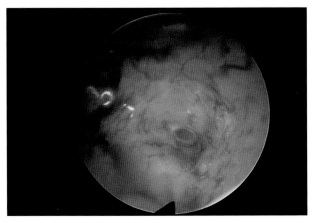

Figure 2.220 Left tubal lumen seen with CO_2.

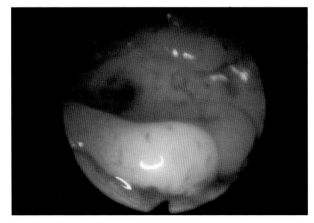

Figure 2.221 Cystic endometrial hyperplasia with large endometrial polyp.

Endometrial abnormalities

Hyperplasia

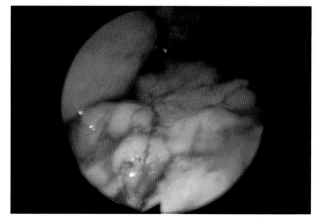

Figure 2.222   Endometrial hyperplasia with multiple polyps.

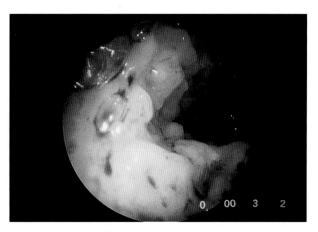

Figure 2.223   Endometrial hyperplasia (courtesy of Milton Goldrath, M.D.).

Polyps

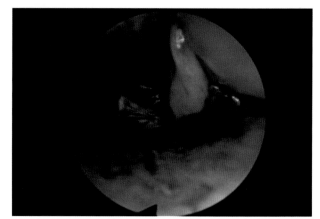

Figure 2.224   Endometrial polyp.

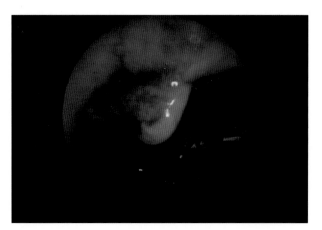

Figure 2.225   Endometrial polyp.

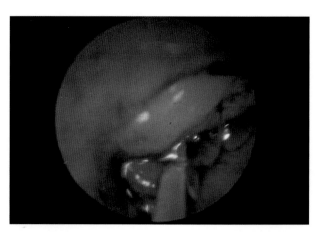

Figure 2.226   Endometrial polyp.

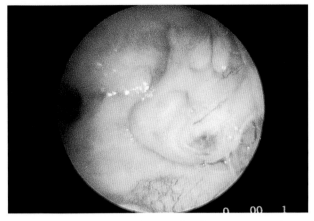

Figure 2.227 Larger endometrial polyp (courtesy of Milton Goldrath, M.D.).

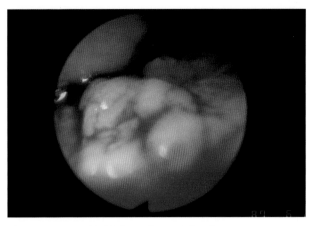

Figure 2.228 Multiple endometrial polyps.

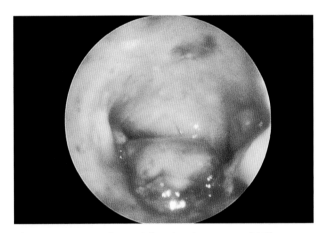

Figure 2.229 Endometrial polyp (courtesy of Milton Goldrath, M.D.).

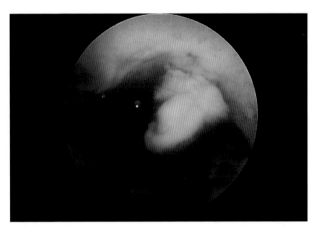

Figure 2.230 Endometrial polyp as seen through Hyskon.

Sub-mucous myomas

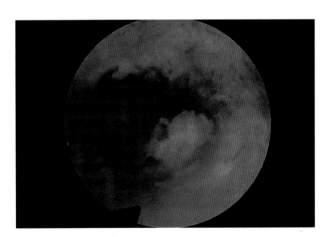

Figure 2.231 Endometrial polyp.

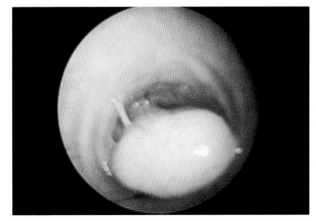

Figure 2.232 Sub-mucous myoma (courtesy of Milton Goldrath, M.D.).

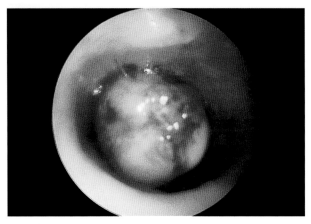

Figure 2.233 Sub-mucous myoma (courtesy of Milton Goldrath, M.D.).

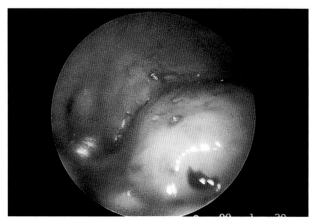

Figure 2.234 Abnormal vasculature of sub-mucous fibroid.

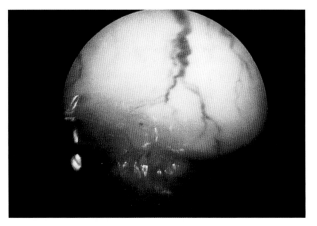

Figure 2.235 Uterine fibroid with abnormal vasculature (courtesy of Milton Goldrath, M.D.).

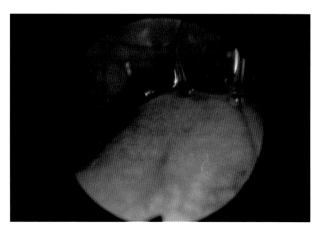

Figure 2.236 Sub-mucous uterine myoma.

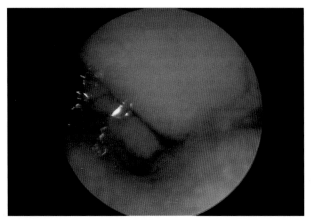

Figure 2.237 Sub-mucous myoma.

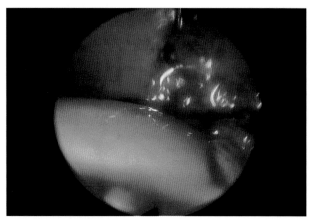

Figure 2.238 Sub-mucous myoma.

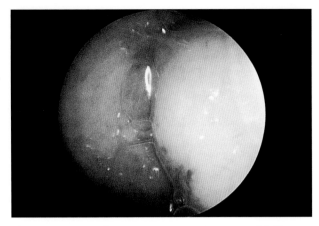

Figure 2.239 Sub-mucous myoma (courtesy of Milton Goldrath, M.D.).

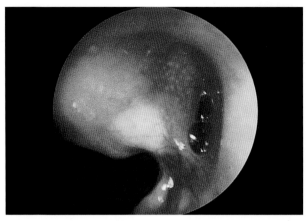

Figure 2.240 Sub-mucous myoma. Often these patients have had multiple dilation and curettages (D&Cs) for bleeding or habitual abortions (courtesy of Milton Goldrath, M.D.).

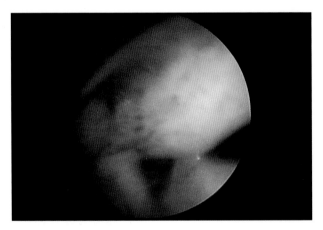

Figure 2.241 Sub-mucous myoma (courtesy of Milton Goldrath, M.D.).

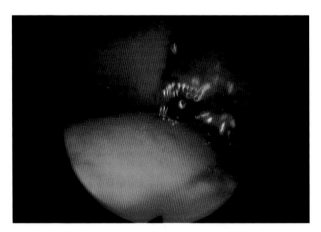

Figure 2.242 Larger sub-mucous myoma.

Intra-uterine adhesions

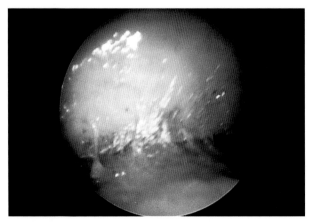

Figure 2.243 Intra-uterine adhesions—Asherman's Syndrome (courtesy of Milton Goldrath, M.D.).

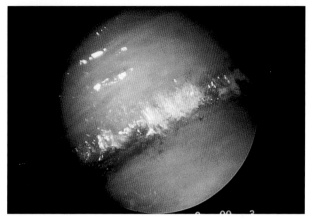

Figure 2.244 Intra-uterine adhesions (courtesy of Milton Goldrath, M.D.).

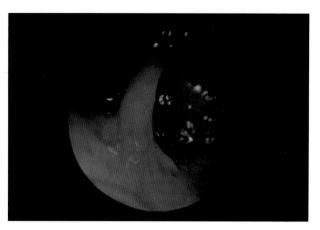

Figure 2.245 More severe uterine adhesions.

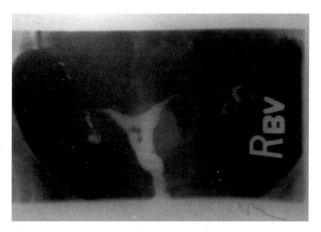

Figure 2.246 Hysterosalpingogram showing intra-uterine defect from Asherman's Syndrome.

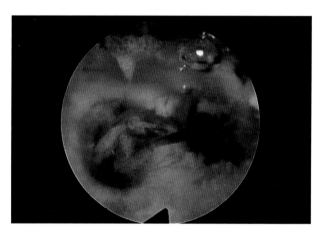

Figure 2.247 Intra-uterine adhesions laterally.

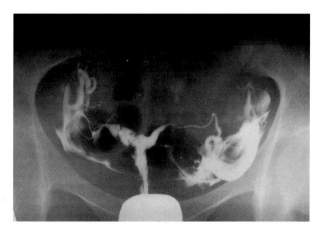

Figure 2.248 Hysterosalpingogram showing adhesions.

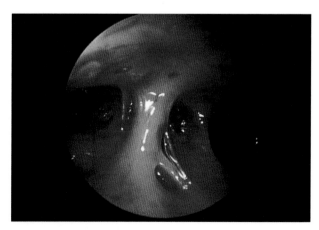

Figure 2.249 Dense intra-uterine adhesions (courtesy of Milton Goldrath, M.D.).

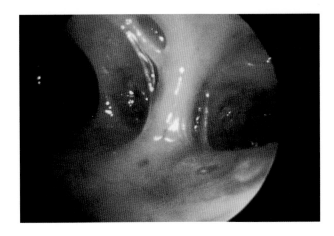

Figure 2.250 Close-up of intra-uterine adhesions (courtesy of Milton Goldrath, M.D.).

Septate uterus

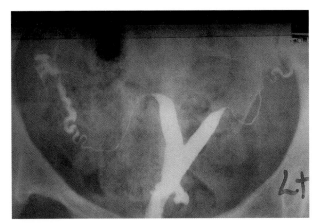

Figure 2.251 Hysterosalpingogram of septate or bicornuate uterus.

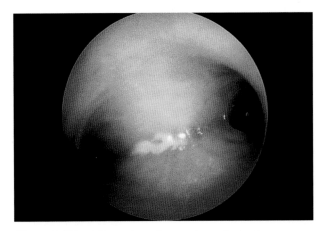

Figure 2.252 View of uterine septum via hysteroscopy (courtesy of Milton Goldrath, M.D.).

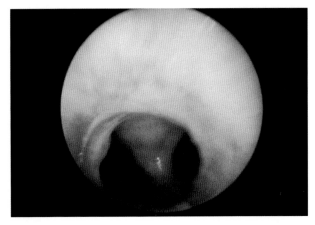

Figure 2.253 Initial view of uterine septum through the cervix.

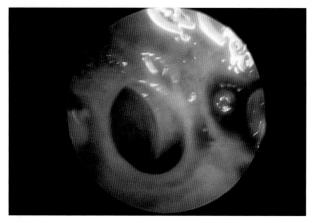

Figure 2.254 Right cornua of septate uterus.

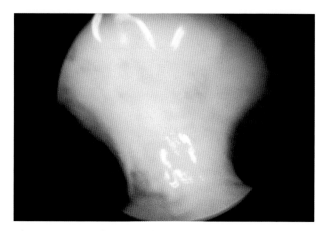

Figure 2.255 Close-up of uterine septum.

Endometrial carcinoma

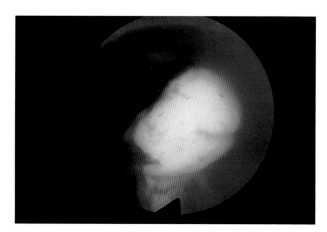

Figure 2.256 Endometrial cancer.

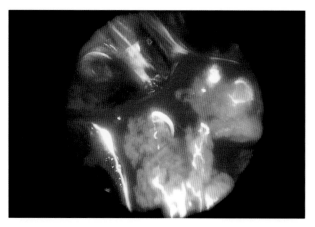

Figure 2.257 Well-differentiated endometrial adenocarcinoma.

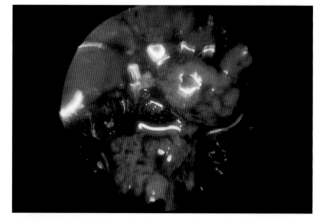

Figure 2.258 Endometrial cancer.

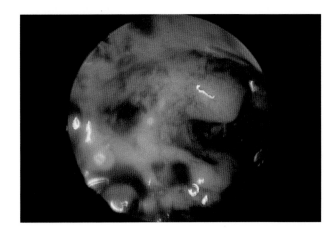

Figure 2.259   Endometrial cancer.

Miscellaneous

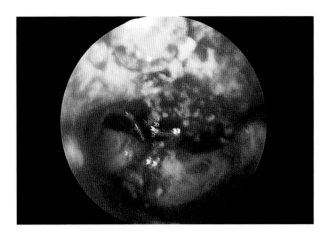

Figure 2.260   Menstrual endometrium.

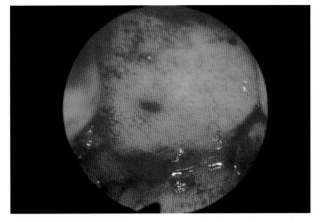

Figure 2.261   Adenomyosis—note the hemorrhagic punctuate area as viewed through the hysteroscope.

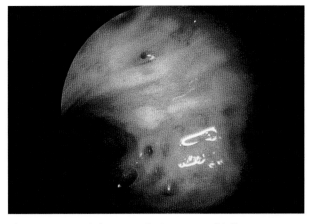

Figure 2.262   Adenomyosis (courtesy of Milton Goldrath, M.D.).

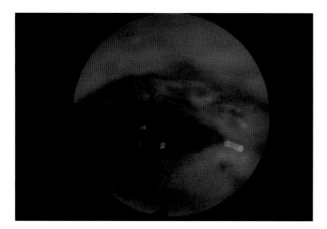

Figure 2.263 Uterine perforation viewed transcervically.

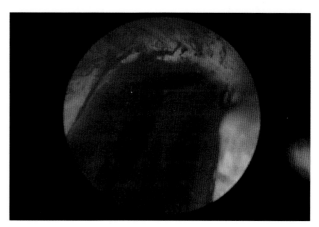

Figure 2.264 Uterine perforation with active hemorrhage.

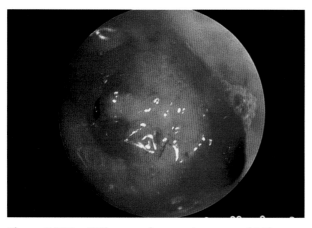

Figure 2.265 DES-exposed uterus (courtesy of Milton Goldrath, M.D.).

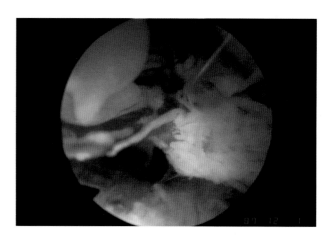

Figure 2.266 A placental polyp seen six weeks after delivery.

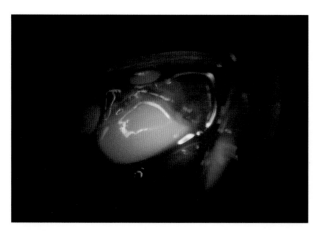

Figure 2.267 Lippes loop IUD.

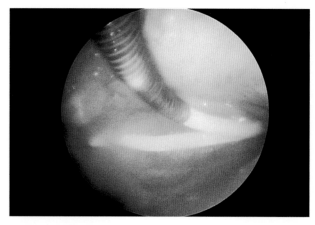

Figure 2.268 Copper-7 IUD (courtesy of Milton Goldrath, M.D.).

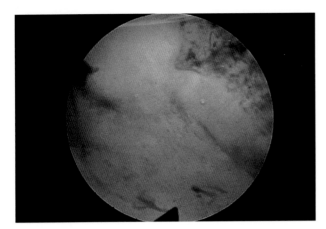

Figure 2.269 Atrophic endometrium.

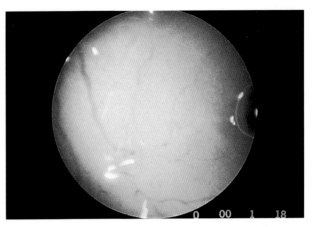

Figure 2.270 Atrophic endometrium (courtesy of Milton Goldrath, M.D.).

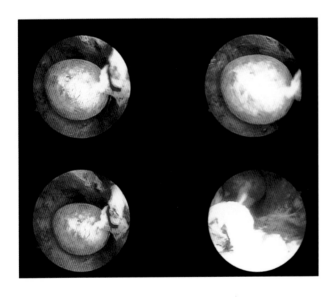

Figure 2.271 Large endometrial polyp caused persistent menometrorrhagia, in spite of attempts of hormonal suppression. The pathology report confirmed early endometrial hyperplasia for this patient who has had long-standing polycystic ovaries documented.

BIBLIOGRAPHY

American Society for Reproductive Medicine: Revised American Society for Reproductive Medicine classification of endometriosis: 1996. *Fertil Steril* **67**:817–21, 1997.

Baggish MS, Barbot J, Valle RF: *Diagnostic and Operative Hysteroscopy, a Text and Atlas.* Chicago, Year Book Medical Publishers, 1989.

Baggish M, Diamond M: Hysteroscopy overview: instrumentation methodology/complications. In: *Contemporary Endoscopy Syllabus for 24th Annual Post-graduate Course.* Birmingham, American Fertility Society, 1991.

Brooks PG: Operative hysteroscopy. In Pitkin RM, Scott JR (eds): *Clinical Obstetrics and Gynecology.* Philadelphia, J.B. Lippincott, Vol. 35, 1992.

Diamond MP: Pelviscopy. In Pitkin RM, Scott JR (eds): *Clinical Obstetrics and Gynecology.* Philadelphia, J.B. Lippincott, Vol. 34, 1992.

Guzick D, Silliman N, Adamson G, et al: Prediction of pregnancy in infertile women based on the American Society for Reproductive Medicine's revised classification of endometriosis. *Fertil Steril* **67**:822–9, 1997.

Johns A: Laparoscopy overview: instrumentation/methodology/complications. In: *Contemporary Endoscopy Syllabus for 24th Annual Post-graduate Course.* Birmingham, American Fertility Society, 1991.

McLaughlin DS (ed): *Lasers in Gynecology.* Philadelphia, J.B. Lippincott, 1991.

McLucas B, Morales AJ, Murphy AA: Endoscopic surgery in gynecology. In: *Current Problems in Obstetrics, Gynecology, and Fertility.* St. Louis, Mosby-Year Book, Vol. 15, 1992.

Semm K, Friedrich ER (eds): *Operative Manual for Endoscopic Abdominal Surgery.* Chicago, Year Book Medical Publishers, 1987.

Siegler AM, Lindemann HJ: *Hysteroscopy Principles and Practice.* Philadelphia, J.B. Lippincott, 1984.

3 Operative procedures

Laparoscopy and hysteroscopy are no longer performed just to establish a diagnosis. Endoscopic treatment of disease states is now a reality due to improved instrumentation and the widespread dissemination of newer technical skills.

Laparoscopic examination of women with chronic pelvic pain revealed endometriosis in 71–83%. The stage and location of endometrial implants do not correlate with the frequency of pelvic pain, including dysmenorrhea and dyspareunia. Every attempt should be made to treat all the pathology completely and restore normal pelvic anatomy in an effort to alleviate pain and/or infertility. Sutton reported that 63% of the patients treated by laser laparoscopy for mild and moderate endometriosis had significant pain relief, as opposed to 23% who had expectant management. Marcoux reported in a randomized, controlled trial that laparoscopic treatment of mild to moderate endometriosis resulted in a cumulative pregnancy rate of 31% versus 18% in the diagnosed, but untreated group.

The laparoscopist should be able to cut, excise, ablate, lyse, coagulate, and vaporize when necessary (Figs 3.1–3.233). As further skills are acquired and mastered, intra-corporeal suturing and knot tying may be learned. The ultimate test of surgical skill is laparoscopic tubal reanastomosis. It has been estimated that 10% of the six million American women who undergo sterilization regret their decision. About 1% wish to restore their fertility by tubal reanastomosis. Sterilization reversal by microsurgical laparotomy had been pioneered by Winston and Gomel twenty years ago. Laparoscopic tubal reversal remains technically challenging (Figs 3.234–3.273), although early published clinical success rates approach 80%. The use of robotic enhancement technology (Zeus, Computer Motion, Inc.), developed specifically to facilitate laparoscopic tubal reanastomosis, aids the surgeon by reducing tremor and fatigue, while adding stability and comfort to the procedure. The first animal survival study has shown a 67% patency rate following the initial use of the Zeus prototype.

The operative hysteroscopist should also be able to ablate, incise, or resect, depending on the pathologic states encountered (Figs 3.274–3.319). The following photographs should aid the operating gynecological endoscopist to improve his or her skills.

Laser pelviscopy

Laser vaporization of endometriosis

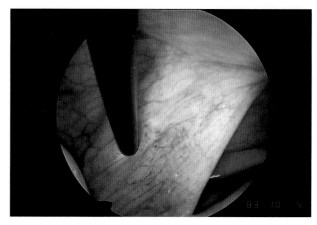

Figure 3.1 Laparoscopic view of peritoneal endometriosis lateral to the left uterosacral ligament.

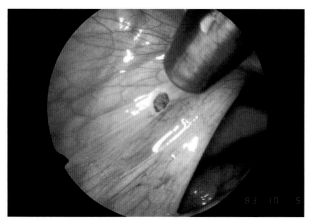

Figure 3.2 CO_2 laser laparoscopy, using a second-puncture probe, is used with a 10 watt non-superpulse as the power setting.

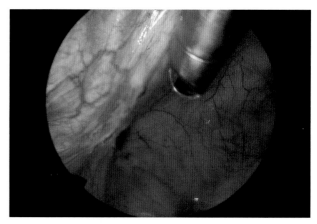

Figure 3.3 Endometriosis is noted inferior to the left ureter. The CO_2 laser beam is reflected off a 45° mirror placed on the second-puncture probe to strike the implant at a 90° angle in order to maximize the power density and minimize the char.

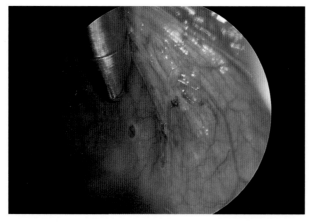

Figure 3.4 Implants of endometriosis vaporized on the right posterior peritoneal surface.

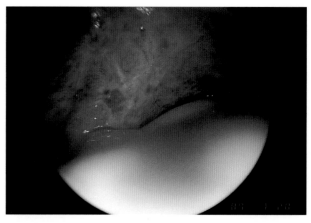

Figure 3.5 Extensive endometriosis stage I prior to vaporization.

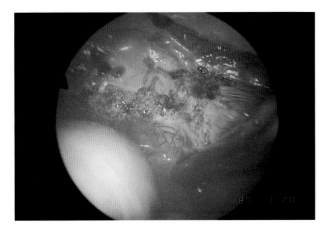

Figure 3.6 Endometriosis stage I status post-vaporization using a 10 watt non-superpulse.

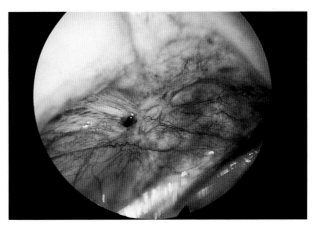

Figure 3.7 Peritoneal implants of endometriosis superior to the left ureter prior to vaporization.

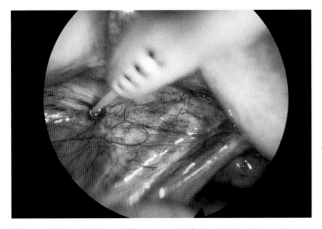

Figure 3.8 A drawn fiber, conical tip (600 microns) with the Nd:YAG laser set at 8 watts is used for partial vaporization of the implants.

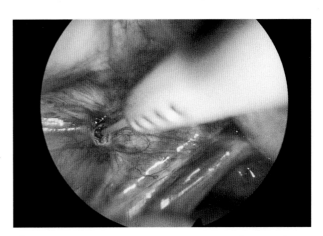

Figure 3.9 An 8 watt power setting is used to continue the vaporization of Fig. 3.10.

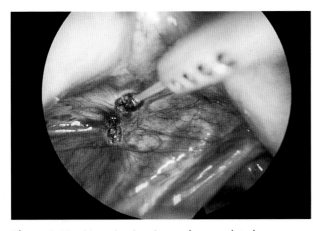

Figure 3.10 Vaporization is nearly completed.

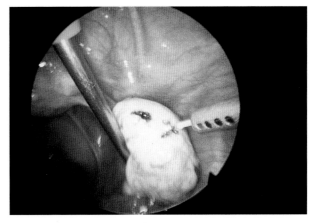

Figure 3.11 Ovarian endometriosis (stage II-A) is seen with the Nd:YAG laser inside the suction-irrigator brought through a second-puncture probe.

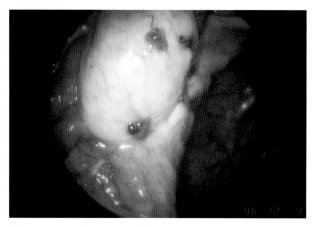

Figure 3.12 Ovarian endometriosis prior to vaporization.

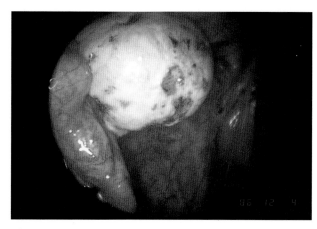

Figure 3.13 Ovarian endometriosis after vaporization using a second-puncture CO_2 laser at 10 watts.

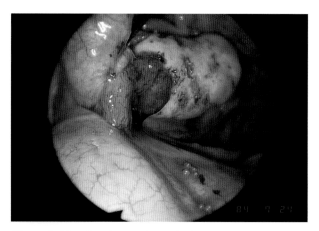

Figure 3.14 Ovarian endometriosis status post-vaporization after irrigation, with heparinized Ringers lactate (1000 units per 1000 cc). Most of the carbon has been removed.

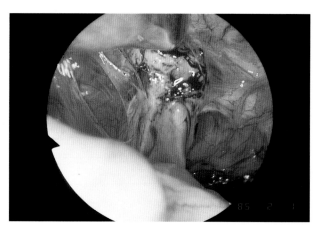

Figure 3.15 Dense adhesions of endometriosis in the posterior cul-de-sac with a fibrous bridge between the rectum and the posterior vagina. Very careful partial vaporization using the CO_2 laser through a second-puncture laparoscope was accomplished at 10 watts.

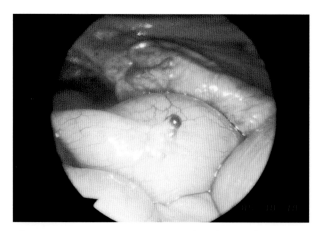

Figure 3.16 Laparoscopic view of surface endometriosis on the serosa of the small bowel.

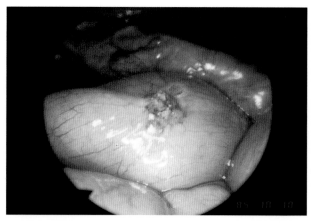

Figure 3.17 Using the interval pulse setting at 5 watts, very careful vaporization was performed through the second-puncture CO_2 laser laparoscope.

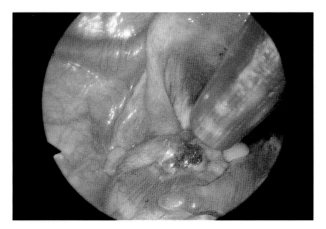

Figure 3.18 Deep implants of endometriosis on the large intestine prior to vaporization.

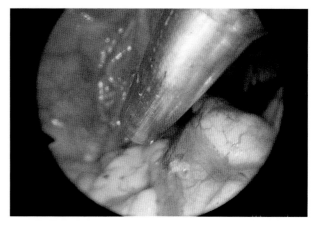

Figure 3.19 Implants noted following partial vaporization. Injecting normal saline through a spinal needle into the serosa of the bowel is helpful to stop the laser's energy from penetrating too deeply.

Laser vaporization of adhesions

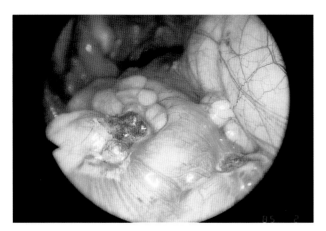

Figure 3.20 Vaporization is nearly completed.

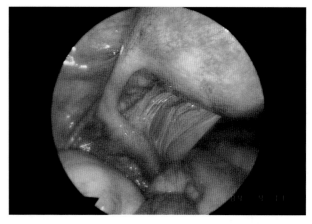

Figure 3.21 Sheets of adhesions separating the ovaries from the fimbria of the tube are noted. This patient had undergone 12 unsuccessful donor inseminations.

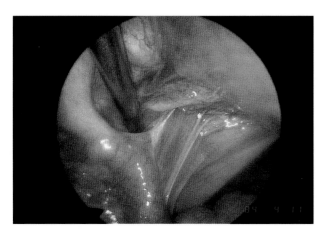

Figure 3.22 Using the CO_2 laser through a second-puncture laparoscope at a 35 watt superpulse, traction is applied.

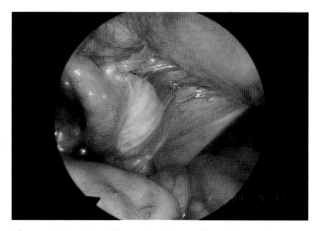

Figure 3.23 Partial vaporization and excision of adhesion is accomplished.

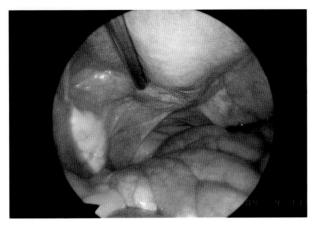

Figure 3.24 The majority of the adhesion is removed.

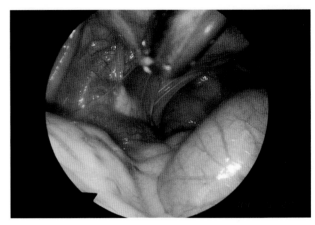

Figure 3.25 This view shows the distal end of the second-puncture CO_2 laser probe.

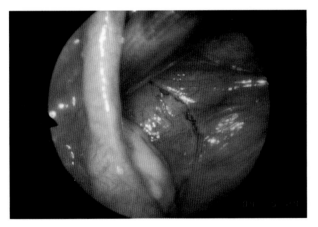

Figure 3.26 The adhesion is completely removed. Note the minimum of carbon debris left behind when the adhesion is totally excised.

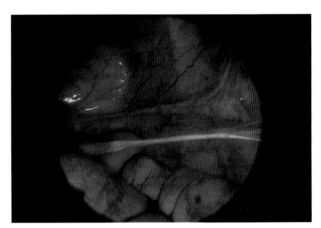

Figure 3.27 An adhesion from the small bowel to the lateral pelvic wall caused intermittent symptoms of bowel obstruction in this patient.

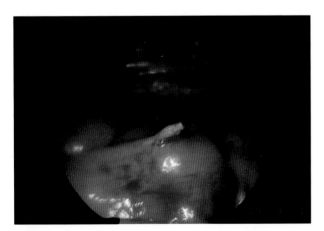

Figure 3.28 Using the single-puncture CO_2 laser laparoscope, at 10 watts of power, the adhesion was vaporized. The peritoneal surface of the lateral pelvic wall was used as a backstop.

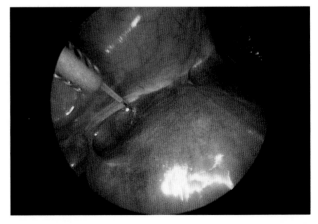

Figure 3.29 A drawn contact fiber (600 micron conical tip), with the Nd:YAG laser set at 8 watts, attacked this adhesion between the uterine fundus and the bladder.

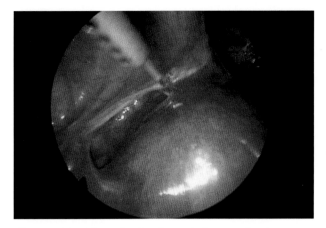

Figure 3.30 The adhesion is partially vaporized.

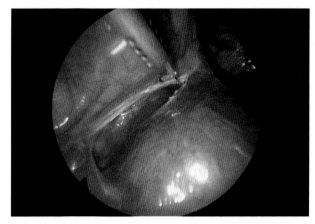

Figure 3.31 The adhesion is partially vaporized. When the tissue is this closely coapted, it is nearly impossible to excise the adhesion.

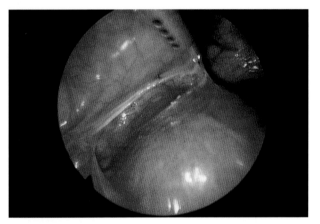

Figure 3.32 The majority of the adhesion has been vaporized. Using traction and counter-traction with the Eder–Cohen uterine cannula as a lever, the laser energy is applied.

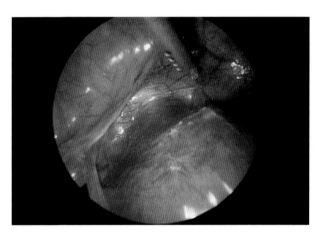

Figure 3.33 The adhesion is nearly completely incised.

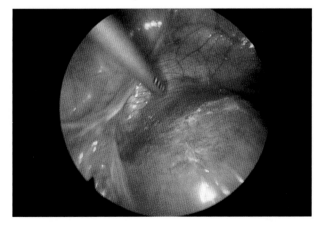

Figure 3.34 The fundal adhesion is completely vaporized, however there remains some lateral pelvic adhesion formation.

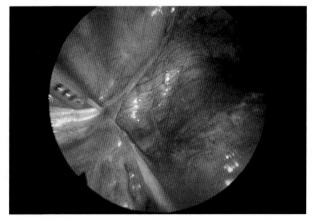

Figure 3.35 The laser set at 35 watts attacks the residual lateral pelvic adhesion.

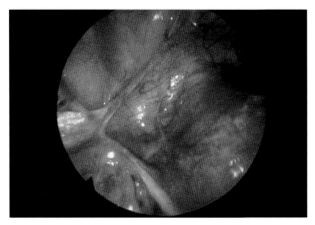

Figure 3.36 Traction and counter-traction facilitate removal of the residual lateral pelvic adhesion.

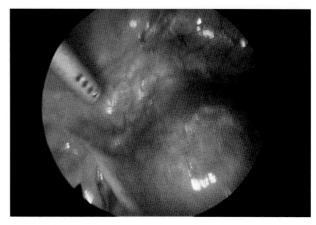

Figure 3.37 The base of the adhesion of Fig. 3.36 is irrigated with heparinized Ringers lactate.

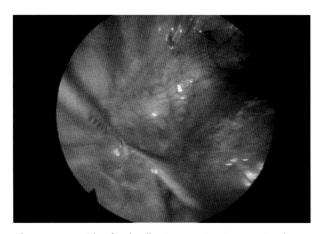

Figure 3.38 The final adhesive portion is vaporized at the conclusion of the procedure.

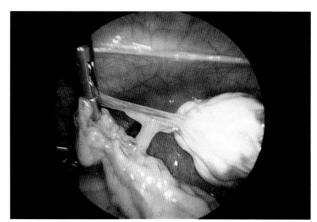

Figure 3.39 A dense adhesion is seen from the right ovary to the small bowel and epiploic fat.

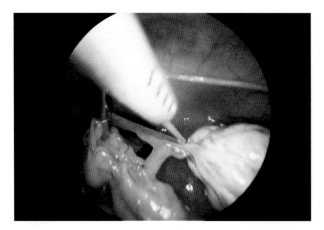

Figure 3.40 Using traction and counter-traction, the Nd:YAG laser is used with a drawn contact fiber, 600 micron conical tip at 8 watts, to incise the adhesion.

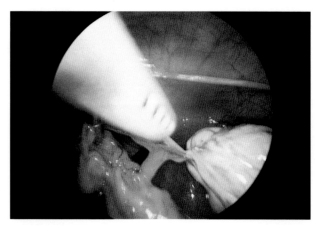

Figure 3.41 The adhesion is partially incised.

Interceed placement

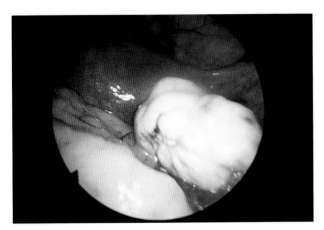

Figure 3.42 The ovary is freed from the dense attachment.

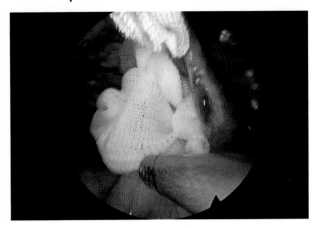

Figure 3.43 Interceed soaked in heparin (1000 units in 10 cc) is placed over the ovary to avoid adhesion reformation to the sidewall.

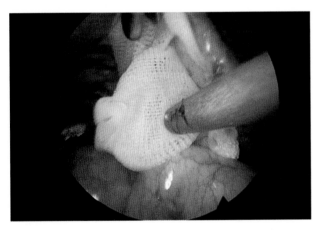

Figure 3.44 Using the graspers from two ports, the Interceed is inserted. Note the lack of bleeding.

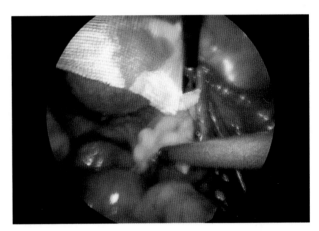

Figure 3.45 The Interceed continues to be spread.

Laser neosalpingostomy

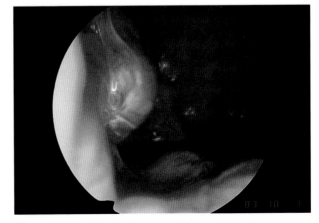

Figure 3.46 The Interceed is finally placed.

Figure 3.47 Distal tubal re-occlusion following micro-surgical neosalpingostomy is seen. The tube is distended transcervically with methylene blue dye.

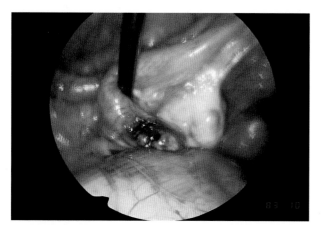

Figure 3.48 The CO$_2$ laser is used at a 35 watts superpulse with a second-puncture probe to incise the distal tube in stellate fashion. The beam is then de-focused at 5 watts to help evert the fimbria.

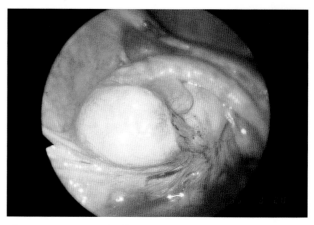

Figure 3.49 Distal tubal re-occlusion is seen in another patient.

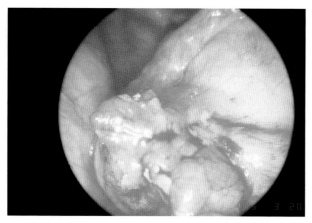

Figure 3.50 Left neosalpingostomy accomplished with the CO$_2$ laser laparoscopic technique at a 35 watt power setting.

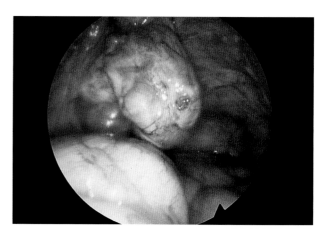

Figure 3.51 Left tubal distal re-occlusion has occurred following neosalpingostomy in this patient.

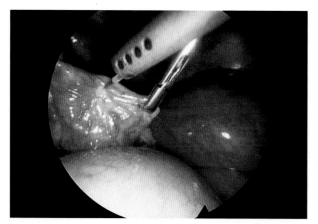

Figure 3.52 Using the Nd:YAG contact drawn fiber, 600 micron conical tip at 8 watts of energy, an incision is made into the tube.

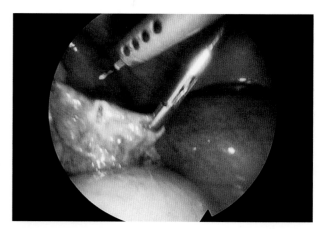

Figure 3.53 Traction and counter-traction are used to continue the incision.

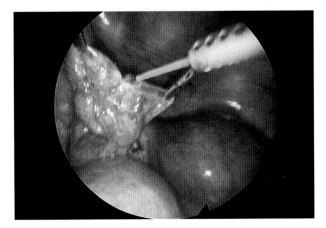

Figure 3.54 The stellate incisions are made.

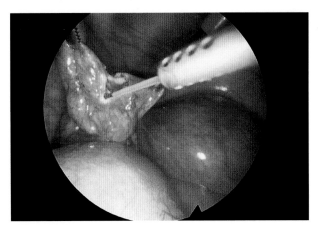

Figure 3.55 The stellate incisions are continued in another direction.

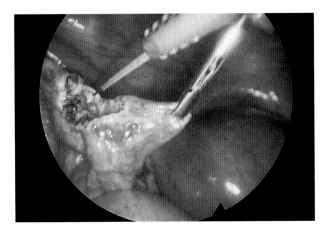

Figure 3.56 The tube is completely opened.

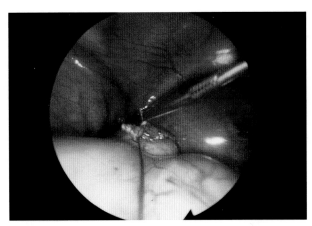

Figure 3.57 Using a 4-0 vicryl, the tube is everted via the pelviscopic suturing technique.

Myomectomy

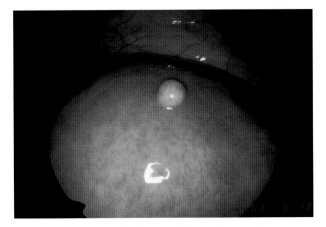

Figure 3.58 A small subserosal fibroid is seen.

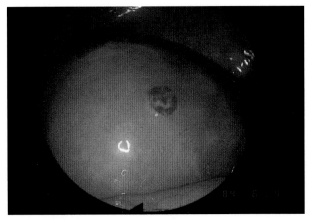

Figure 3.59 Using 35 watts superpulse with the CO_2 laser second-puncture probe, the area is vaporized directly.

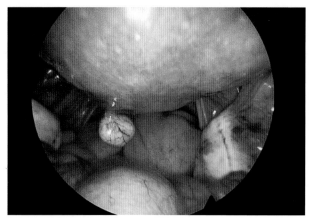

Figure 3.60 A small subserosal fibroid is noted on the posterior wall of the uterus.

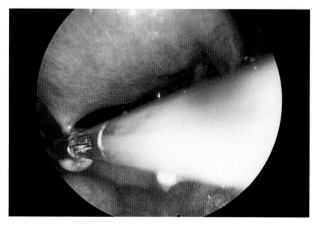

Figure 3.61 The fibroid is grasped through the operating channel with a single-puncture laparoscope.

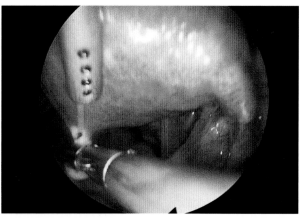

Figure 3.62 The Nd:YAG laser contact fiber is used at 8 watts to incise the base.

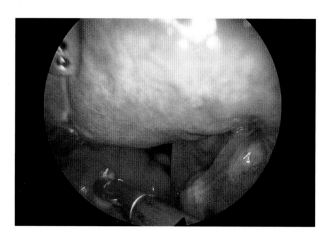

Figure 3.63 The fibroid is excised.

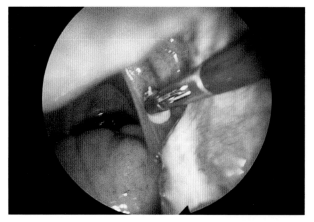

Figure 3.64 The fibroid is brought through the operating channel of the single-puncture laparoscope.

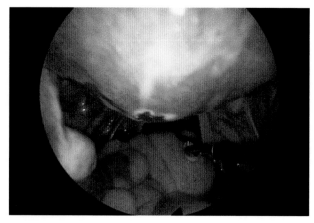

Figure 3.65 The base of the myoma is cauterized to control bleeding.

Laser LUNA (laparoscopic uterosacral nerve ablation)

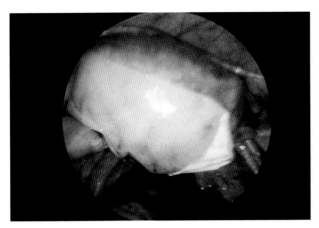

Figure 3.66   In another patient treated by microlaser myomectomy a Gore-Tex® patch has been placed over the defect and viewed six weeks later via second-look laparoscopy.

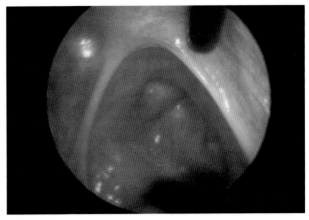

Figure 3.67   Laparoscopic uterosacral nerve ablation (LUNA) may be accomplished to relieve dysmenorrhea. This is usually done if no other pathology is seen.

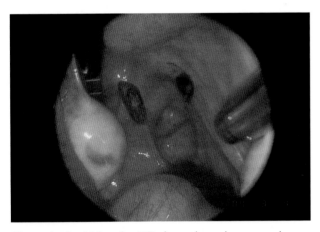

Figure 3.68   Using the CO_2 laser through a second-puncture probe at 10 watts superpulse, the uterosacral ligament is transected. With traction and counter-traction via the Eder-Cohen cannula, an elliptical defect is made.

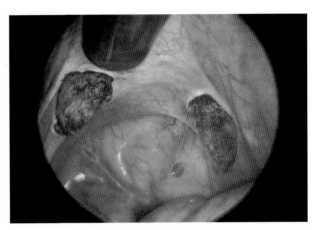

Figure 3.69   Note the absence of bleeding if the incision is made more medially.

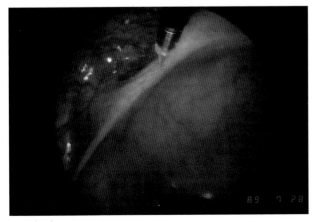

Figure 3.70   The LUNA may be done with a conical sapphire Nd:YAG tip.

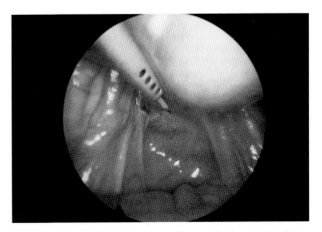

Figure 3.71   A drawn contact fiber with the Nd:YAG is used to make the LUNA.

Laser decompression of polycystic ovaries

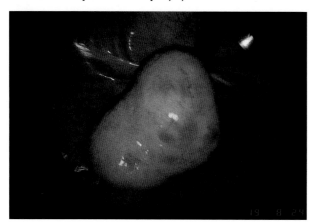

Figure 3.72 Polycystic ovaries as viewed through the laparoscope.

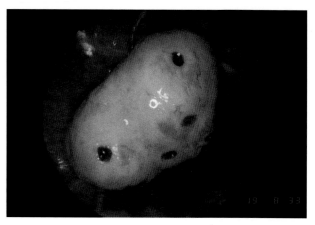

Figure 3.73 Using the CO_2 laser through a single-puncture operating channel at 35 watts superpulse, the cysts are systematically decompressed.

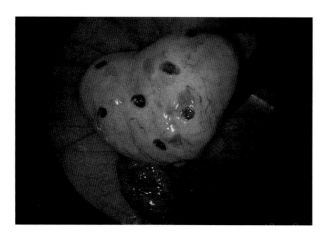

Figure 3.74 Note the completion of the polycystic ovarian decompression. It is very important to use high power settings at superpulse to avoid charring the tissue with subsequent adhesion formation.

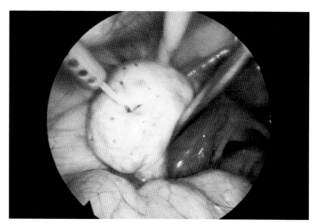

Figure 3.75 The fiber lasers are better to perform this procedure, as seen with the Nd:YAG contact fiber. The micro-Bovi tip may be used as well.

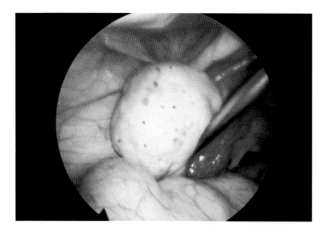

Figure 3.76 Completion of the decompression of the polycystic ovaries. Recent data indicate that this technique normalizes ovarian function resulting in stable androgen production for 18–20 years.

Salpingo-oophorectomy with an intact uterus using endoloops

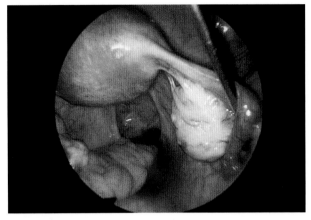

Figure 3.77 Tubal ovarian adhesions may be treated with the Nd:YAG laser.

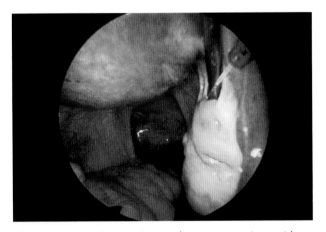

Figure 3.78 Using traction and counter-traction, with a conical tip contact fiber at 8 watts, the adhesion is approached.

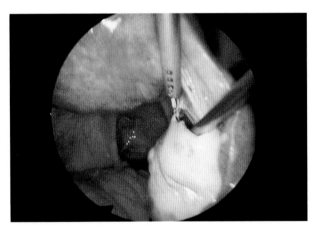

Figure 3.79 The adhesion is partially vaporized.

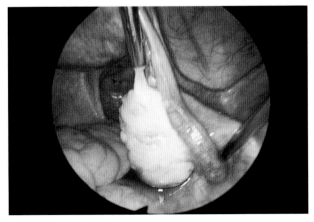

Figure 3.80 Using bipolar cautery the utero-ovarian ligament is cauterized and then divided.

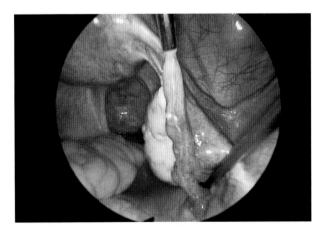

Figure 3.81 The tube is cauterized and divided with the plan to endoscopically remove the right tube and ovary.

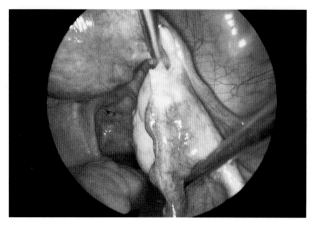

Figure 3.82 Completion of the tubal cautery.

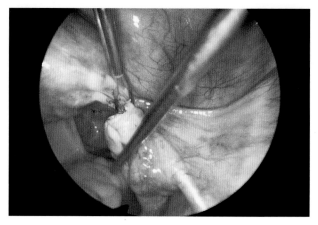

Figure 3.83 The tube and ovary are grasped.

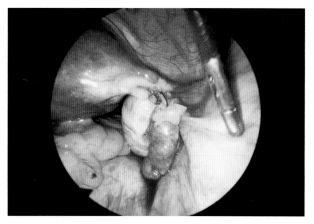

Figure 3.84 The tube and ovary are free from their attachment to the uterus.

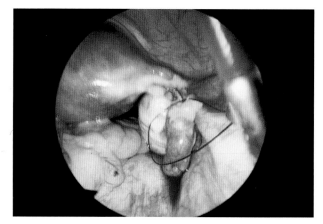

Figure 3.85 The 0-PDS endoloop is placed next to the tube and ovary.

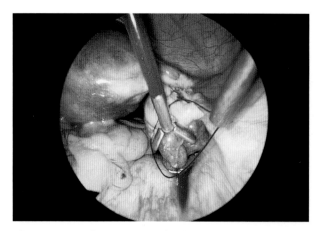

Figure 3.86 The grasper grabs the tube and ovary.

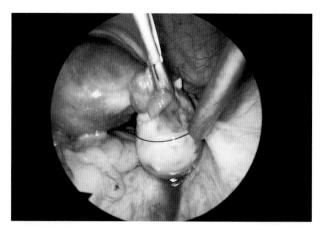

Figure 3.87 The endoloop is placed around the adnexa.

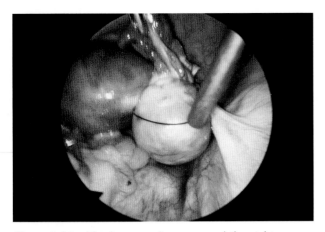

Figure 3.88 The loop continues around the right adnexa with an ovarian cyst.

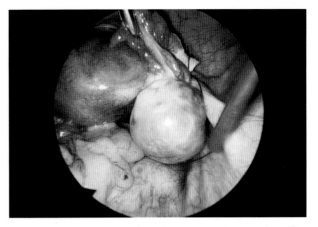

Figure 3.89 Care must be taken to avoid entangling the small bowel as the loop is continued around the adnexa.

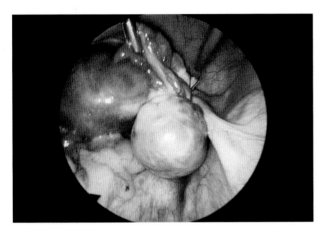

Figure 3.90 The knot pusher pushes the knot tight to strangulate the tissue.

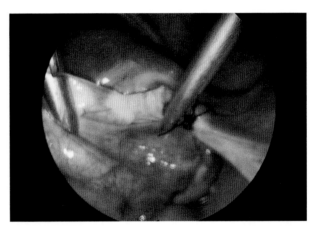

Figure 3.91 The tube and ovary are grasped from the central lower trocar and the scissors are used to begin to excise the tube and ovary.

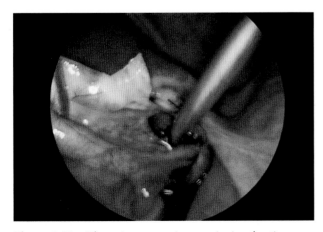

Figure 3.92 The scissors continue to incise the tissue.

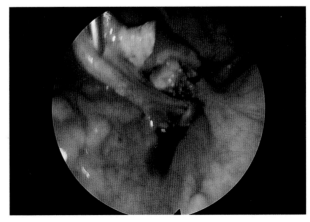

Figure 3.93 The adnexa is pulled away from the vascular pedicle with traction.

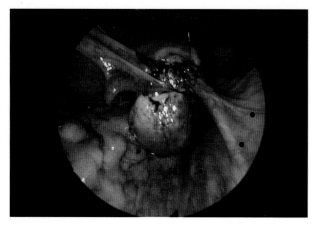

Figure 3.94   The tube is removed.

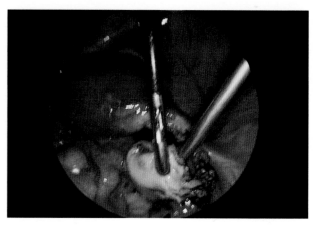

Figure 3.95   The ovary is grasped with a grasper and the scissors are used to cut through the ovarian vascular attachment.

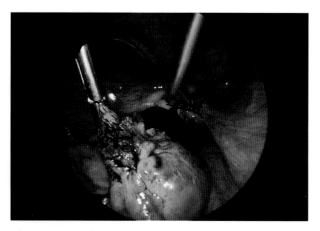

Figure 3.96   The ovary with the cyst is grasped through the 5 mm central trocar with a grasper.

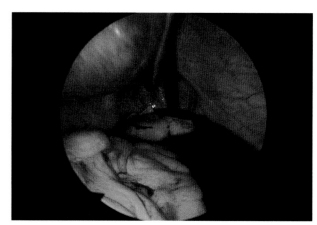

Figure 3.97   The adnexa is placed in the posterior cul-de-sac.

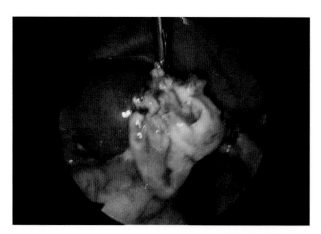

Figure 3.98   The adnexa is grasped with the grasper through the right lower second-puncture trocar as the single-puncture operating laparoscope is placed through the umbilical incision.

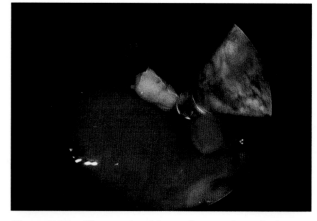

Figure 3.99   The ovarian biopsy forceps through the operating laparoscope grasps the ovary.

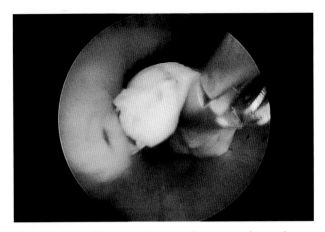

Figure 3.100 The ovary is partially retracted into the sheath, decompressing the cyst, as the tube and ovary are wrestled through the umbilical incision, and grasped externally with a hemostat.

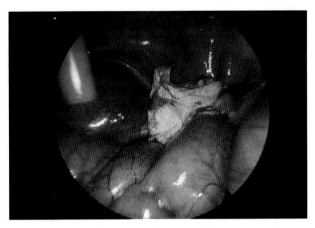

Figure 3.101 The 10 mm diagnostic laparoscope is replaced as Interceed is draped over the pedicle.

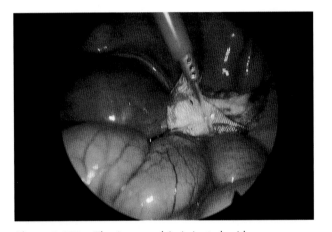

Figure 3.102 The Interceed is irrigated with heparinized Ringers lactate (1000 units per 10 cc).

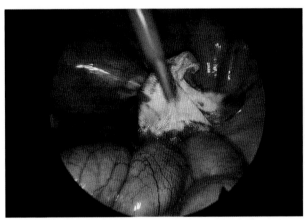

Figure 3.103 The Interceed is placed tightly on the pedicle.

Salpingo-oophorectomy of residual ovaries using endoloops

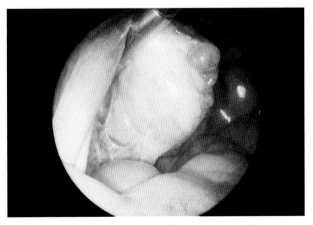

Figure 3.104 Removing a residual ovary may be difficult due to the dense adhesions to the lateral pelvic wall.

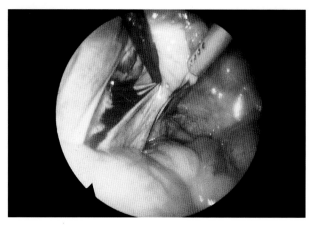

Figure 3.105 Lateral pelvic wall adhesions are elevated with probes as the contact Nd:YAG laser is brought in through a right second-puncture trocar.

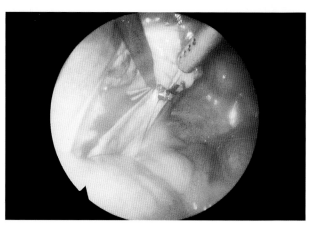

Figure 3.106 Using 8 watts with a drawn fiber, the lateral pelvic wall adhesions are very carefully vaporized after identifying the ureter.

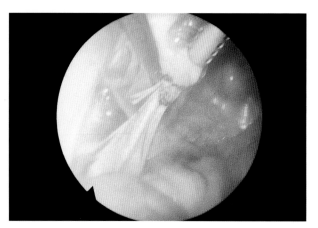

Figure 3.107 Some smoke production is apparent during vaporization, which may begin to obscure the operating field and needs to be evacuated.

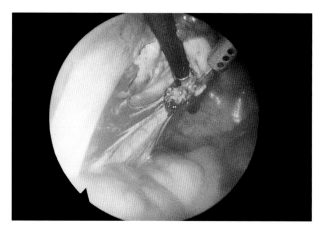

Figure 3.108 The tube and ovary continue to be retracted away from the lateral pelvic wall as the adhesion is attacked by the Nd:YAG laser.

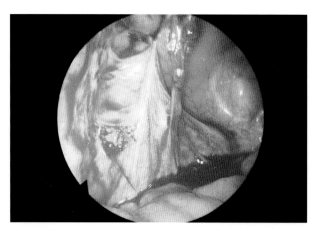

Figure 3.109 The tube and ovary are free of its attachments as an endoloop is placed.

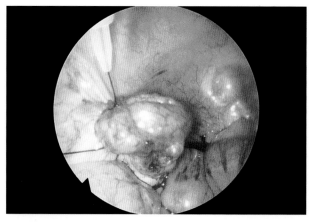

Figure 3.110 The endoloop has strangulated the adnexal blood supply.

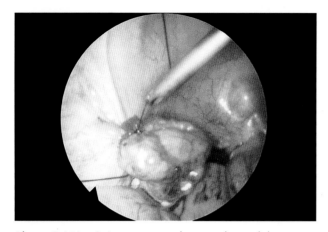

Figure 3.111   Scissors are used to cut the endoloops.

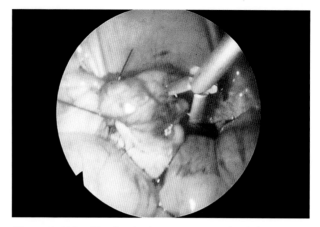

Figure 3.112   The hooked grasper is used to obtain a firm hold on the adnexa.

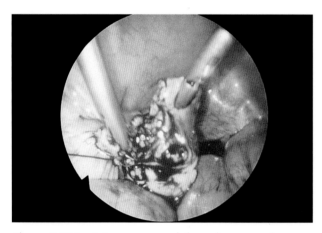

Figure 3.113   Scissors are used through a second-puncture trocar to excise the tube and ovary from the lateral pelvic wall.

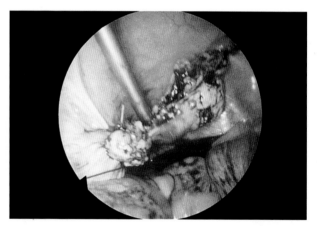

Figure 3.114   The adnexa is nearly completely removed.

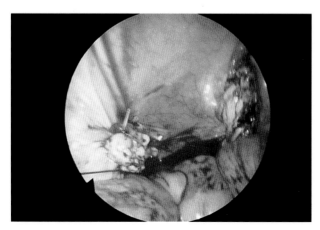

Figure 3.115   The adnexa is totally removed showing the strangulated blood supply. It is then removed through the single-puncture laparoscope.

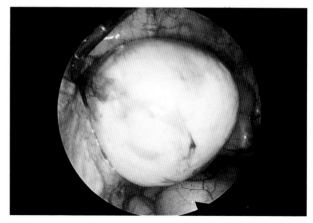

Figure 3.116   A left residual ovary is seen with a recurrent ovarian cyst which causes pain.

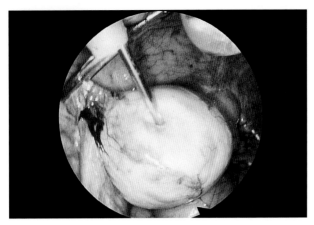

Figure 3.117 A needle is placed into the cyst to aspirate the fluid. It is sent to cytology if the adnexa is to remain or discarded if the adnexa is to be removed (as in this case).

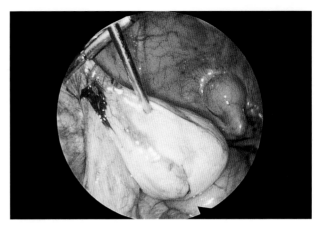

Figure 3.118 The ovary is nearly collapsed, which will facilitate pelviscopic removal.

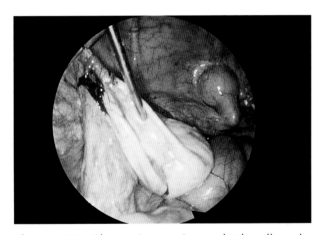

Figure 3.119 The ovarian cyst is completely collapsed.

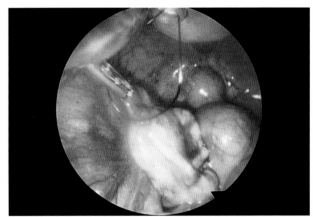

Figure 3.120 The endoloop is placed near the adnexa through a second-puncture trocar.

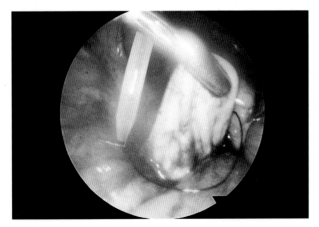

Figure 3.121 The ovary is grasped and the loop encircles it.

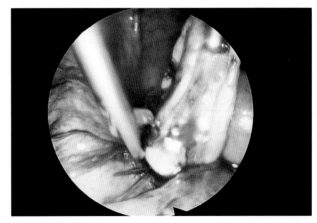

Figure 3.122 The knot is pushed down to strangulate the blood supply.

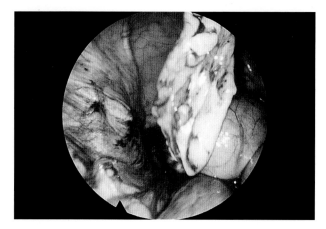

Figure 3.123 The ovary is excised with scissors.

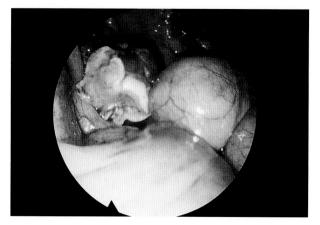

Figure 3.124 Interceed is placed over the base of the pedicle.

Endosuture of peritoneal defect

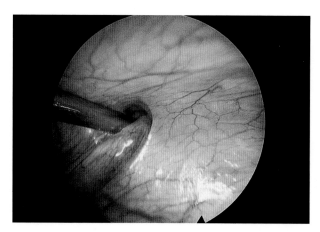

Figure 3.125 A small hernia is noted as the right round ligament traverses through the abdominal wall.

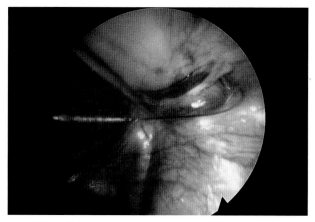

Figure 3.126 Using 4-0 nylon with a straight needle, the peritoneal edges are approximated.

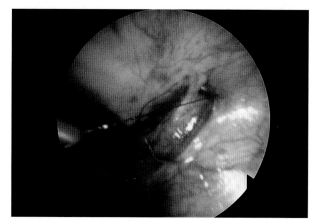

Figure 3.127 Peritoneal edges are tied intra-abdominally.

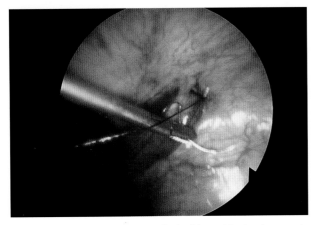

Figure 3.128 Note the needle holder with the free end.

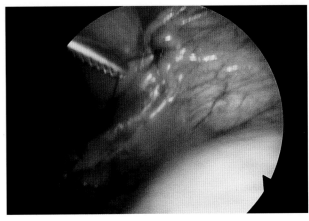

Figure 3.129 The knot is continued and cinched down.

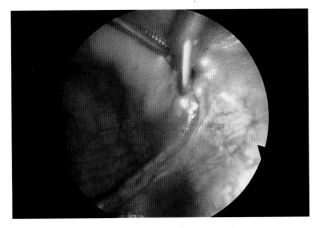

Figure 3.130 Scissors remove the remaining suture material.

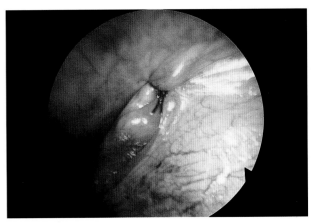

Figure 3.131 The hernia is closed as the procedure is completed.

Salpingo-oophorectomy with endoscopic linear cutter

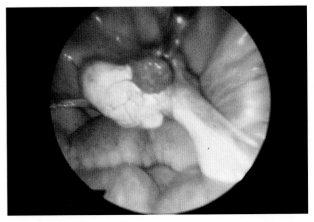

Figure 3.132 To remove the right tube and ovary, the ovarian pedicle is grasped and elevated.

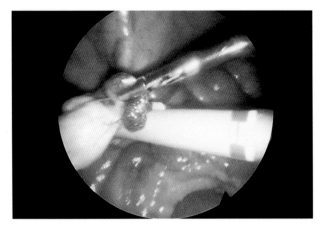

Figure 3.133 The tissue thickness is gauged; it is determined that a blue cartridge is needed for the multi-fire endoscopic gastrointestinal anastomosis (GIA).

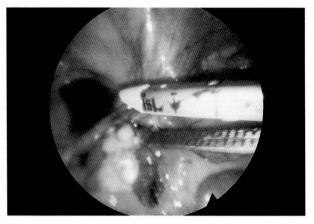

Figure 3.134 The multi-fire endoscopic GIA is placed with the gray lever on the handle externally opened to open the jaws of the instrument intra-abdominally.

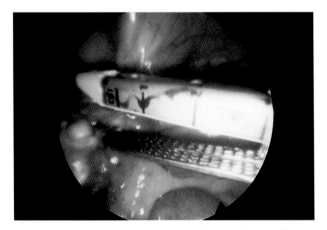

Figure 3.135 Note the markings which delineate the length of the staple line.

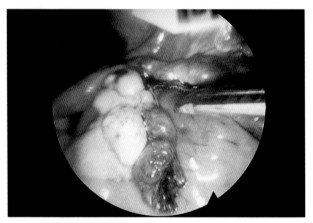

Figure 3.136 The jaws have been closed, the endoscopic GIA fired, and the jaws re-opened to show the staple line where the tissue has been transected.

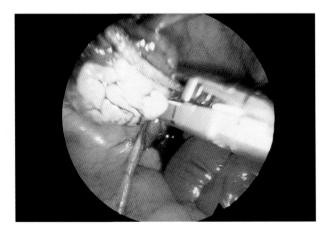

Figure 3.137 The staple line is more apparent on the adnexa as another bite is taken with the endoscopic GIA after refilling the cartridge.

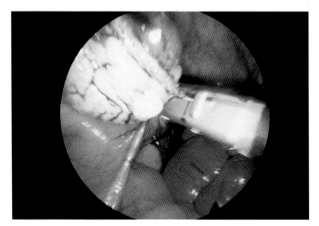

Figure 3.138 The jaws are closed.

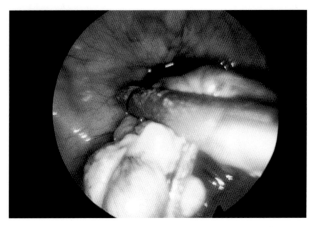

Figure 3.139 The tissue is assessed anteriorly and posteriorly to be sure that the staple lines will go far enough without injuring any surrounding structures.

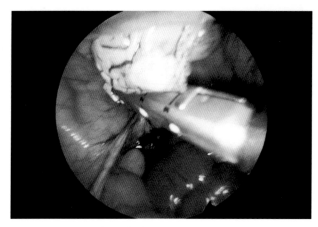

Figure 3.140 Inferiorly there appears to be no unwanted tissue in the jaws.

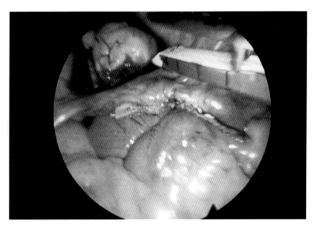

Figure 3.141 The endoscopic GIA has been fired and the adnexa seen detached. Note the hemostatic suture line.

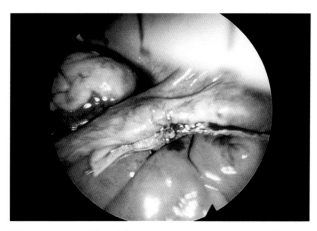

Figure 3.142 The right tube and ovary are placed in the anterior cul-de-sac awaiting removal through the single-puncture laparoscope. An alternate method uses a 5 mm laparoscope through a second-puncture trocar and the 10 mm large grasper is placed through the umbilical trocar for tissue removal.

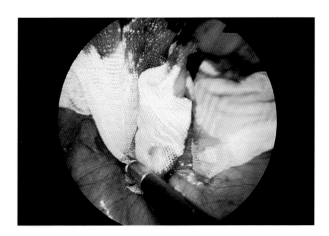

Figure 3.143 Interceed is placed over the pedicle on the lateral pelvic wall.

Endoscopic appendectomy

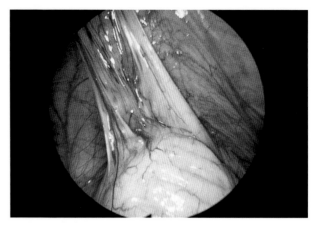

Figure 3.144   Dense bowel adhesions are noted from the colon to the right anterior abdominal wall.

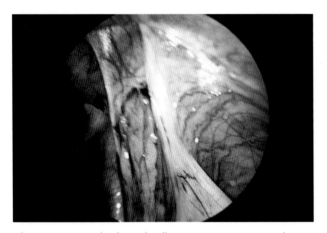

Figure 3.145   The bowel adhesions appear to involve the tip of the appendix. A central second-puncture probe is placed.

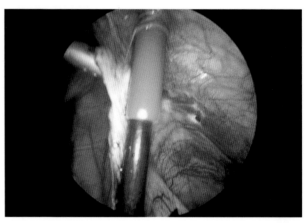

Figure 3.146   Very carefully, a right lateral probe is placed away from the adhesion.

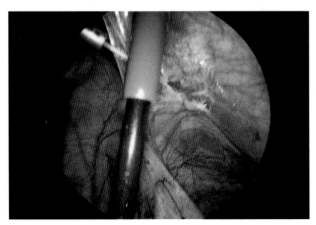

Figure 3.147   The contact Nd:YAG laser fiber is used at 8 watts to begin to incise the adhesions and mobilize the cecum.

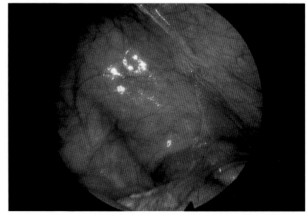

Figure 3.148   The cecum has been mobilized from its attachments.

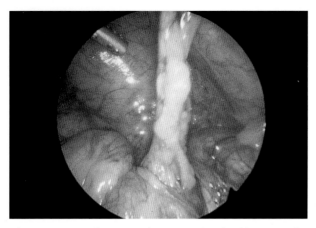

Figure 3.149 The appendix is noted to be fibrotic and has been freed from the abdominal wall.

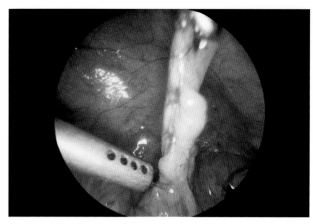

Figure 3.150 The meso-appendix is vaporized with the laser.

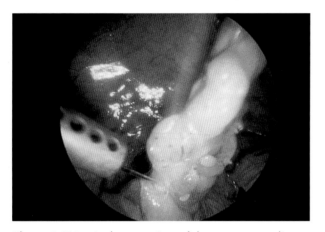

Figure 3.151 A close-up view of the meso-appendix.

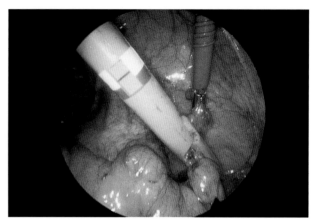

Figure 3.152 The tissue thickness gauge is placed; a white cartridge is needed.

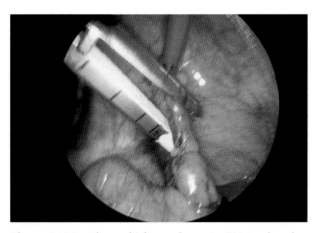

Figure 3.153 The multi-fire endoscopic GIA is placed into the abdominal cavity and the jaws are opened.

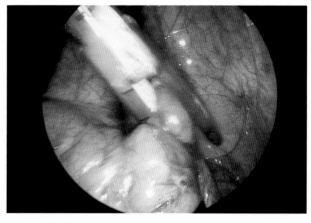

Figure 3.154 The jaws are placed around the base of the appendix and closed.

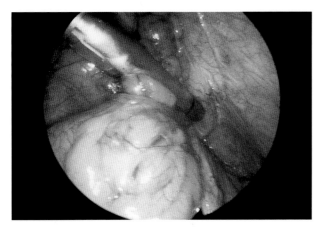

Figure 3.155 The endoscopic GIA is fired.

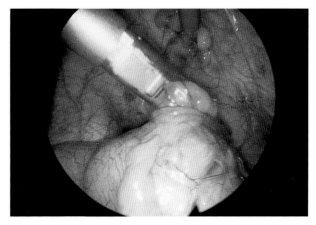

Figure 3.156 Most of the base of the appendix has been incised.

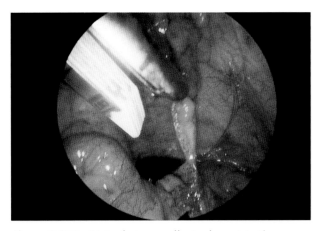

Figure 3.157 Note that a small attachment to the cecum remains as the multi-fire endoscopic GIA is removed.

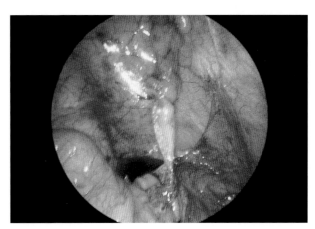

Figure 3.158 An endoloop is placed around the tip of the appendix for traction.

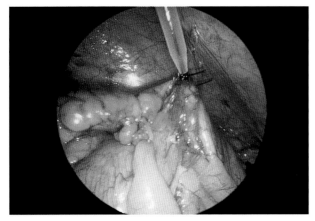

Figure 3.159 Three endoloops are placed at the base of the appendix using 0-PDS to finish the appendectomy.

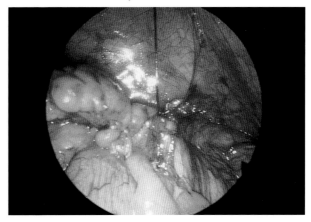

Figure 3.160 The endoloop prior to cutting.

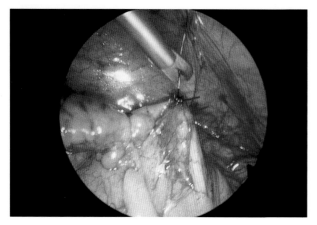

Figure 3.161 The endoloop is cut.

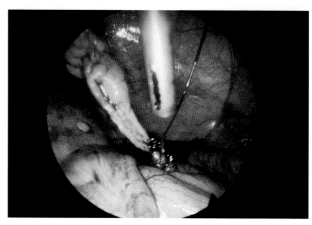

Figure 3.162 The remaining portion of the base of the appendix is incised with the laser and the appendix is removed.

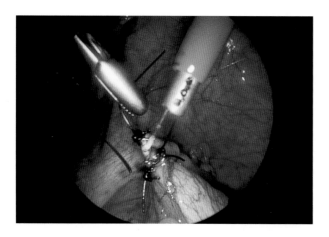

Figure 3.163 The base is irrigated profusely with heparinized Ringers lactate.

Laser linear salpingostomy for ectopic pregnancy

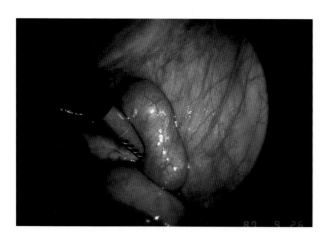

Figure 3.164 A mid-segment unruptured right ectopic pregnancy has been diagnosed. The implantation sites occur: 75% in the ampulla; 12% in the isthmus; 5% in the fimbria; 2% in the cornua; and 3% in the abdominal, ovarian or cervical sites. In selected patients, systemic methotrexate has resulted in outcomes similar to laparoscopic salpingostomy with regard to subsequent pregnancy and tubal patency. However, medical therapy has resulted in a negative impact on health-related quality of life, which may be due to the prolonged treatment with methotrexate and persistence of the ectopic pregnancy. Laparoscopic salpingostomy, therefore, should not be replaced by methotrexate therapy, unless an informed choice is made by the patient after being fully educated regarding the side effects.

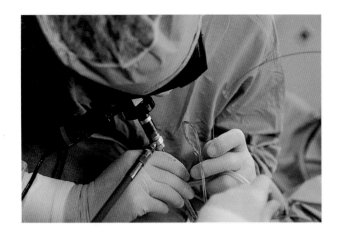

Figure 3.165 A fiber laser is most helpful in removing the ectopic pregnancy hemostaticly. An initial quantitative beta human chorionic gonadotropin (beta-hCG) reading is obtained on day 35 and repeated 48 hours later. If there is less than a 66% rise and vaginal ultrasound has not shown an intra-uterine gestational sac, diagnostic laparoscopy is pursued at about day 42–45. Usually the implantation site is visualized if the beta-hCG reading is greater than 2000 mIU.

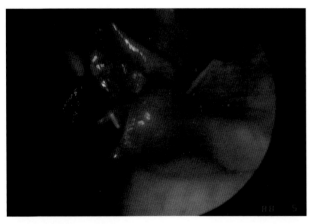

Figure 3.166 Using the argon laser, a small incision is made over the ectopic. The incision does not need to be as long as the ectopic pregnancy as usually the tissue may be teased out. The author finds it helpful to add 10 units of pitocin to the intravenous line to help the tube contract and expel the products of conception.

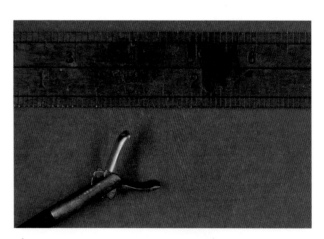

Figure 3.167 A 3 mm grasper is used.

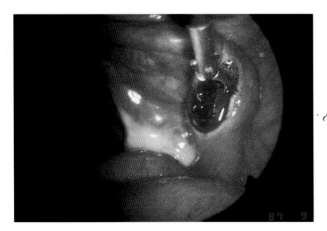

Figure 3.168 The grasper helps to dilate the implantation site and extract the products of conception.

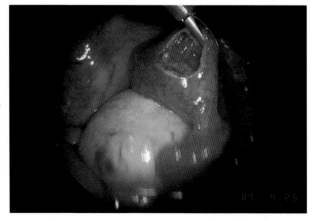

Figure 3.169 The implantation site is irrigated. Hemostasis is controlled with unipolar fine point cautery as needed.

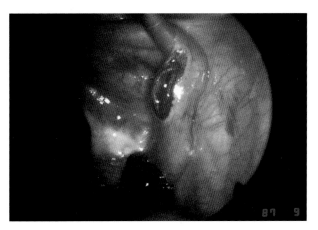

Figure 3.170 The ectopic is placed in an accessible spot to facilitate removal by the 10 mm cup device.

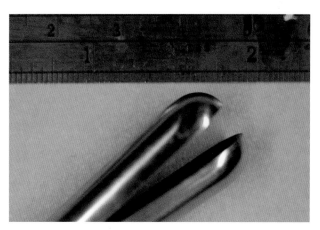

Figure 3.171 The cup device is placed through the 10 mm infra-umbilical trocar.

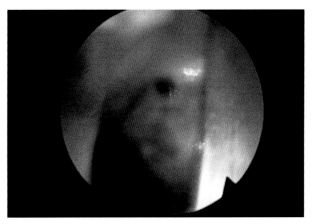

Figure 3.172 Note the view through a second-puncture 5 mm laparoscope showing the ectopic pregnancy inside the cup, which is then removed.

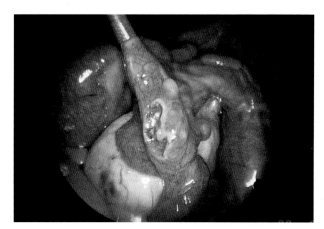

Figure 3.173 The 10 mm diagnostic laparoscope is placed sub-umbilically to check for hemostasis.

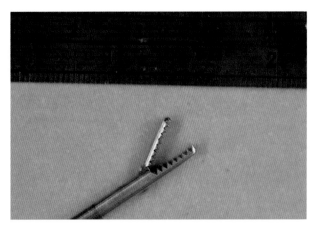

Figure 3.174 A 3 mm needle holder is helpful to suture the site if so desired.

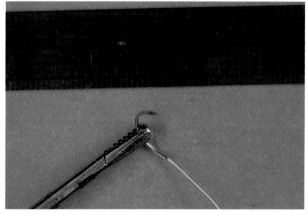

Figure 3.175 Usually a curved needle enables coaptation of the serosal edges, which is infrequently regained.

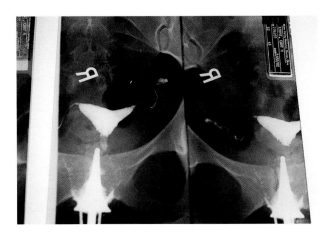

Figure 3.176 A hysterosalpingogram is usually performed after six months to confirm tubal patency. The patient is warned immediately post-operatively regarding the chance of a chronic ectopic pregnancy (about 5% incidence). Quantitative beta-hCG readings are obtained weekly until less than 5 mIU. The patient is admitted overnight and the hemoglobin rechecked in the morning. Should the beta-hCG plateau or rise, methyltrexate or salpingectomy would be advised. Conservative laparoscopic treatment is recommended if the ectopic pregnancy is less than 3 cm, unruptured, and the patient desires to retain her reproductive potential.

Salpingectomy for ectopic pregnancy

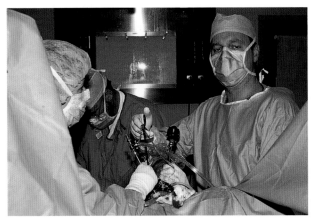

Figure 3.177 Definitive surgical therapy, i.e. laparoscopic salpingectomy, is advised for tubal rupture, overt hemorrhage anatomic distortion, and/or if further pregnancy is not desired.

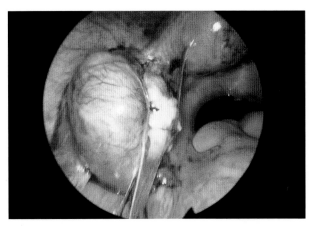

Figure 3.178 This patient's ectopic pregnancy involves the majority of the tube with marked tubal dilatation where previous adhesion formation has occurred.

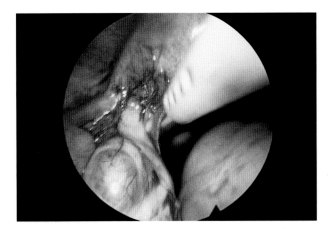

Figure 3.179 The contact YAG laser is brought in through the right lower quadrant and, at 8 watts, the adhesions are vaporized.

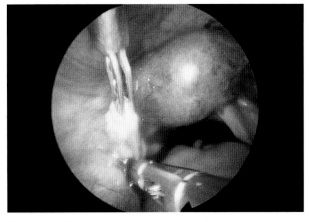

Figure 3.180 A bipolar cautery is used to coagulate the proximal portion of the tube.

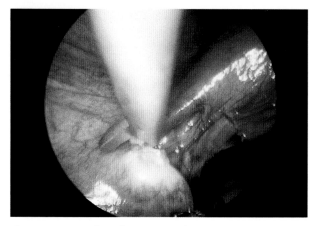

Figure 3.181   The tube is incised.

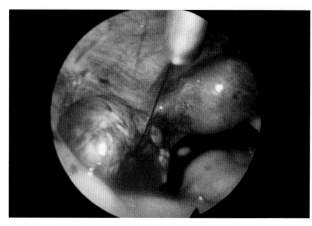

Figure 3.182   An endoloop is placed around the tube.

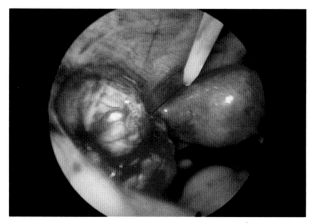

Figure 3.183   The knot pusher is withdrawn after the tissue has been strangulated.

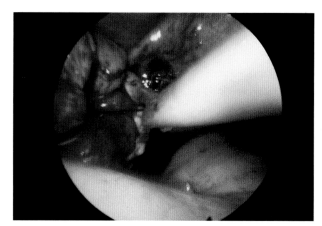

Figure 3.184   The suture is cut.

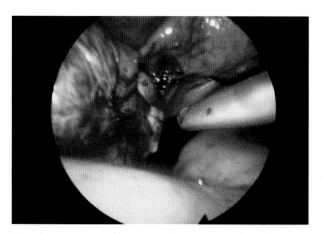

Figure 3.185   Another two endoloops are placed and the suture cut.

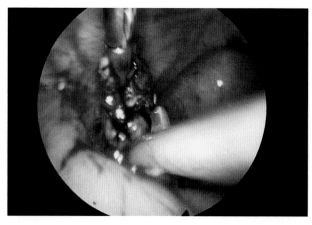

Figure 3.186   The tube is excised by the scissors using traction.

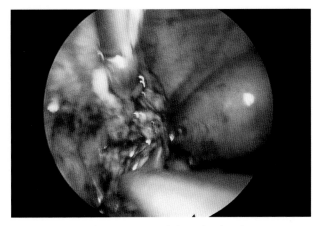

Figure 3.187 The majority of the tube has been excised.

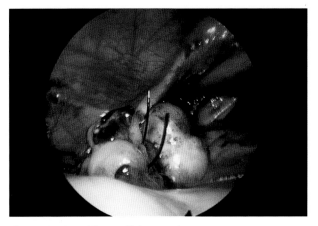

Figure 3.188 The pedicle remains.

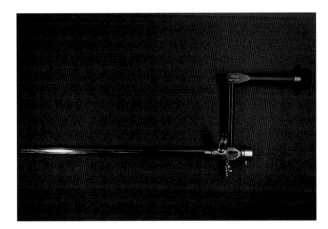

Figure 3.189 The single-puncture laparoscope with its 8 mm operating channel is used to remove the tubal pregnancy.

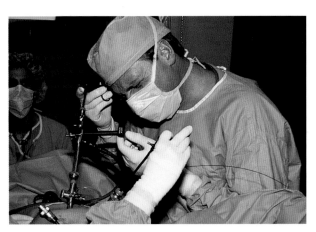

Figure 3.190 The laparoscope is placed through the umbilical incision with a hooked grasper placed through the operating channel.

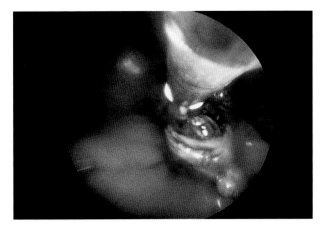

Figure 3.191 Note the view of the hooked grasper holding the tubal pregnancy. It is important to grasp the distal end to avoid milking the tubal pregnancy out as the tube is removed.

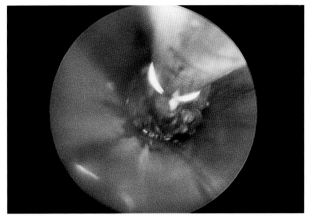

Figure 3.192 The tubal pregnancy is brought into the operating channel of the laparoscope.

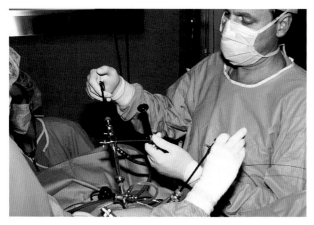

Figure 3.193 The grasper, the laparoscope, and the tubal pregnancy are rotated through the abdominal wall.

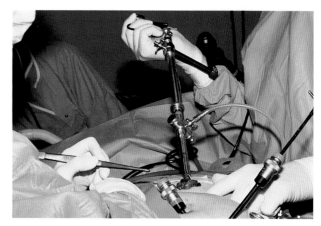

Figure 3.194 The tube is grasped by the assistant with a hemostat as it exits the abdominal cavity.

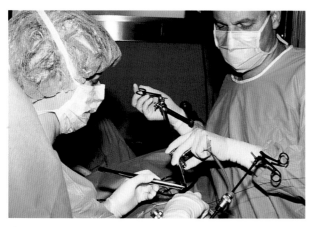

Figure 3.195 The ectopic pregnancy is removed intact.

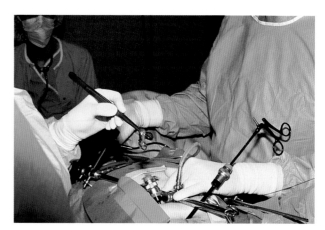

Figure 3.196 The specimen is passed off.

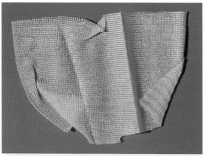

Figure 3.197 Interceed is soaked in heparin (1000 units in 10 cc).

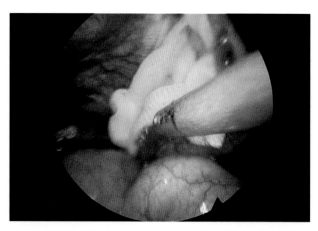

Figure 3.198 The Interceed is put through the central 12 mm trocar and placed over the pedicle.

Removal of abdominal (ovarian) ectopic pregnancy

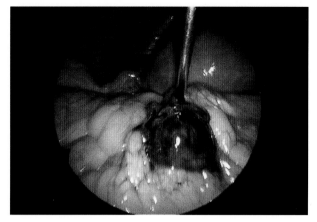

Figure 3.199   An abdominal ectopic pregnancy is noted probably following a tubal abortion onto the omentum.

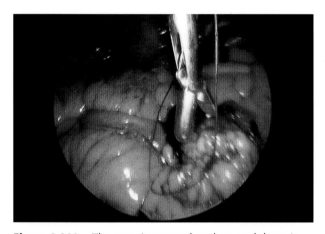

Figure 3.200   The area is grasped and an endoloop is placed.

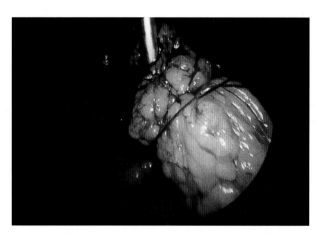

Figure 3.201   The tissue is bunched with the endoloops.

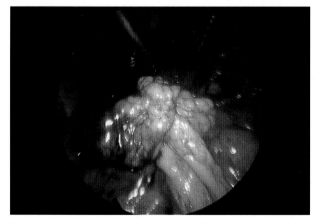

Figure 3.202   Three endoloops are placed to strangulate the tissue.

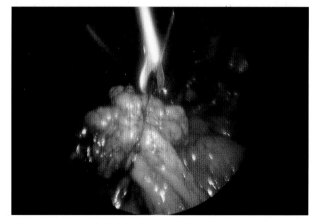

Figure 3.203   The sutures are cut.

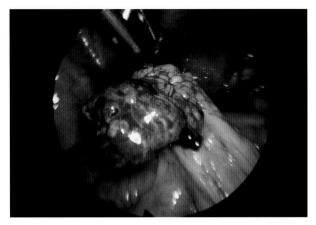

Figure 3.204 The abdominal ectopic pregnancy is strangulated.

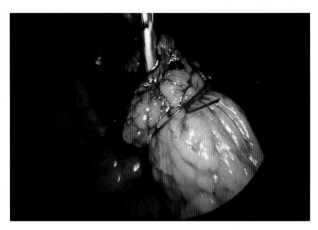

Figure 3.205 The ectopic is excised.

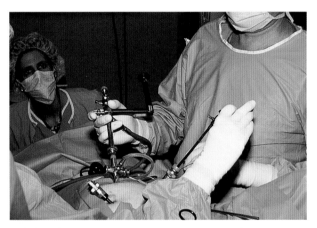

Figure 3.206 The ectopic is brought through the abdominal wall by single-puncture laparoscope.

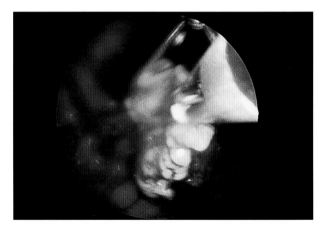

Figure 3.207 Note the endoscopic view of the ovarian ectopic.

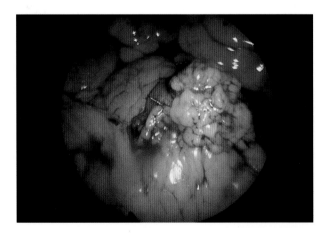

Figure 3.208 Note the omentum following removal of the ovarian ectopic.

Removal of Gore-Tex® patch

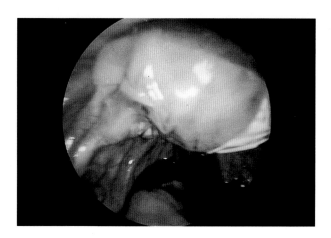

Figure 3.209   Early second-look laparoscopy shows a Gore-Tex® patch which had been previously placed over a large myomectomy scar and left lateral pelvic wall following microlaser laparotomy. Multiple myomectomies and extensive adhesiolysis between the rectum and the uterus had been performed. Note the absence of adhesion reoccurrence.

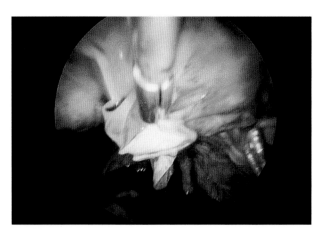

Figure 3.210   A permanent (Surgilon) anchor suture in the mid-portion of the fundus is removed in order to peel the Gore-Tex® off the uterus.

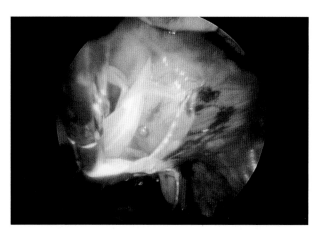

Figure 3.211   Minimal bleeding is encountered as the patch is removed.

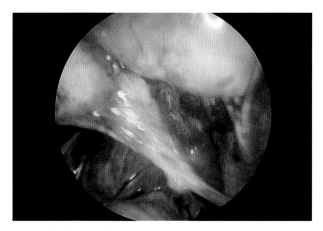

Figure 3.212   A fibrous exudate is usually present beneath the patch; this is removed as well.

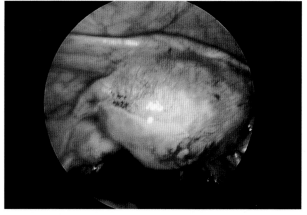

Figure 3.213   Note the minimal bleeding which occurs with patch removal along with the marked improvement in restoring normal pelvic anatomy following the previous microlaser surgery.

Pelviscopic removal of hydrosalpinges prior to IVF

Figure 3.214 Vandromme et al published that hydrosalpinges had an adverse effect on the success of IVF (*Human Reprod* **10**:576, 1995). They reported an increase from 10%/retrieval to 38%/retrieval following tubal repair or salpingectomy. This patient had previously been treated conservatively for her five ectopics, and had an early missed Ab following her first IVF cycle, elsewhere. Bilateral salpingectomy was advised and performed prior to her next IVF cycle, which resulted in the birth of twins. This laparoscopic view shows the hydrosalpinges being endolooped.

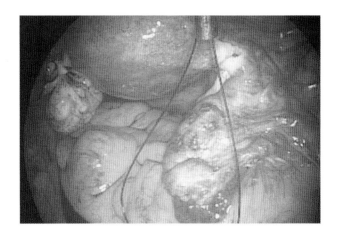

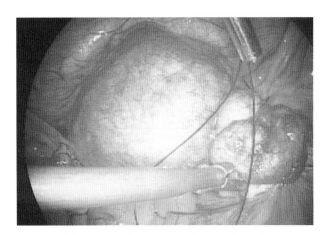

Figure 3.215 The tube is grasped through the loop.

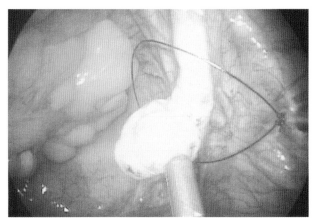

Figure 3.216 The loop is moved toward the cornua.

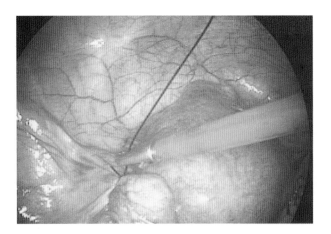

Figure 3.217 The loop is cinched, strangulating the blood supply, then the tube is excised and removed through the umbilical trocar site.

Contact laser fibers

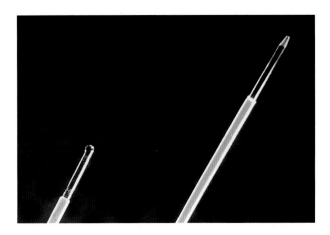

Figure 3.218 The contact laser fibers, ball tipped and conical, which may be used in conjunction with the Diode, KTP, Nd:YAG, and Argon lasers. The energy is concentrated in the conical tip for precise incision of adhesions and cysts, while the energy is dispersed through the ball tip for endometriosis (courtesy of Laser Peripherals).

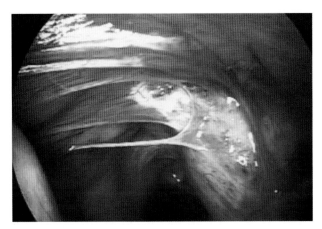

Figure 3.219 When discovered, one should be prepared to treat adhesions, but the backstop should be known in order to avoid vital intra-abdominal structures.

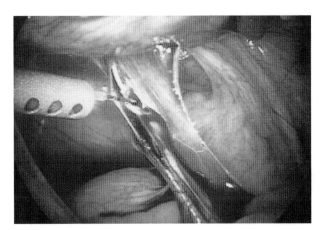

Figure 3.220 The conical tipped laser fiber is used with the Diode laser, at 6 watts, to evaporate this adhesion. Traction and counter-traction are helpful to minimize the thermal spread of laser energy as well as to facilitate the removal of the adhesion.

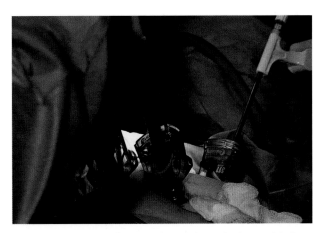

Figure 3.221 The fiber is placed through the Reddick–Saye suction-irrigator, which has a guide channel for the laser fiber. This helps stabilize the fiber to enhance the precision of the application of the laser energy.

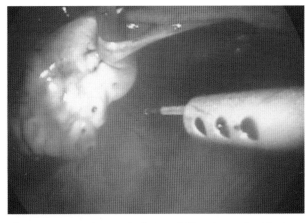

Figure 3.222 The conical tipped fiber is used with the same laser energy to decompress subcapsular cysts for those patients with polycystic ovaries.

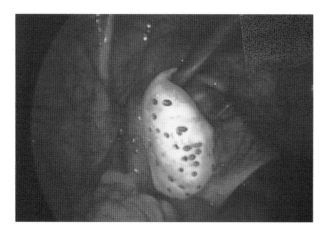

Figure 3.223 When the procedure is completed, it appears as if a track shoe had walked on the surface of the ovary. Subsequent adhesions are rare if there is minimal spread of thermal energy. Using low-power CO_2 laser settings or high-power Bovie coagulation settings may result in adnexal adhesions, and care should be taken to avoid this complication.

LAVH

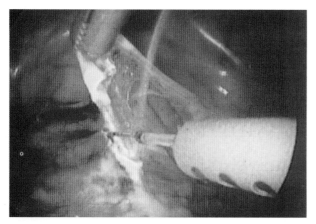

Figure 3.224 For laparoscopic assisted vaginal hysterectomy (LAVH), after the pelvic pathology and the course of the ureters are assessed, the Diode laser is used with a conical tipped fiber, at 6 watts, to incise the posterior then anterior peritoneum. This step facilitates safe vaginal entry to complete the procedure.

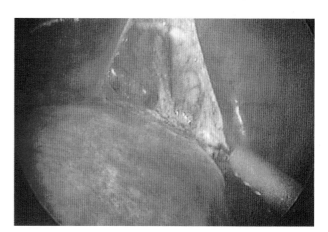

Figure 3.225 Using bladder traction anteriorly, the peritoneal reflection is mobilized away from the uterus.

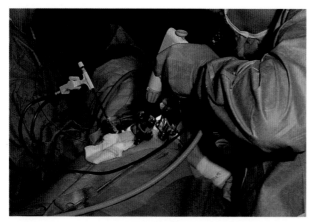

Figure 3.226 The multi-fire endoscopic GIA is placed through the 12 mm umbilical port, viewing the pelvis through a 10 mm laparoscope place left of the umbilicus.

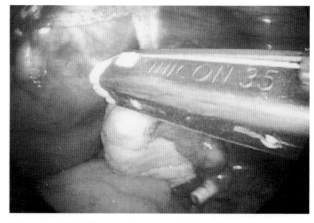

Figure 3.227 The endoscopic GIA is placed into the abdominal cavity.

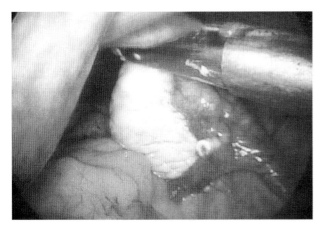

Figure 3.228 The tissue is grasped with the endoscopic GIA, which is then fired, and the tissue is divided between two rows of staples.

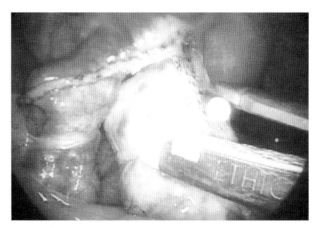

Figure 3.229 The jaws are released, and the tissue cut confirmed.

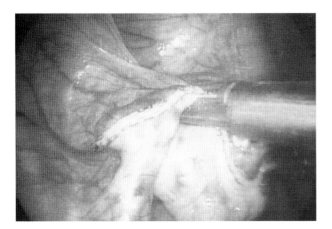

Figure 2.230 The next area of tissue to be stapled is subsequently grasped, divided, and stapled. Usually, three to four areas are stapled on each side of the uterus, stopping short of the uterine arteries, in order to reduce the chance of ureteral damage. Prior to tissue stapling, it is a good habit to confirm, again, the course of the ureter on the side of tissue stapling.

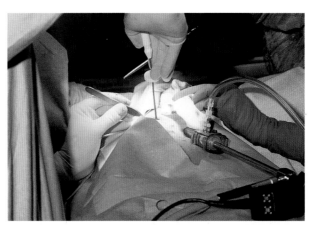

Figure 3.231 The 10 mm trocar site, left of the umbilicus, is closed by inserting the Endojudge, with a 2-0 vicryl reel attached, to facilitate fascial closure. The laparoscope is inserted umbilically to confirm the trocar site closure without including a loop of bowel.

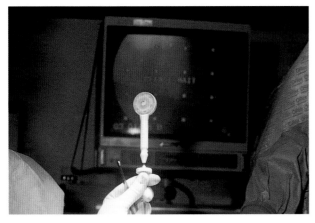

Figure 3.232 The Endojudge may be used without direct visualization, as experience is gained.

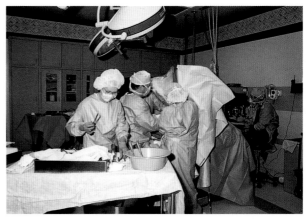

Figure 3.233 The remainder of the LAVH is performed using standard surgical techniques.

Laparoscopic microsurgical tubal reanastomosis

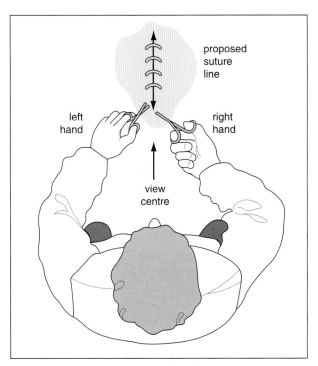

Figure 3.234 The most technically challenging technique of pelviscopy is laparoscopic microsurgical tubal reanastomosis. It is helpful, when trying to master this technique, to try to duplicate the same approach laparoscopically as one does with the open technique. (Figs 3.286–3.293 and 3.308–3.325 taken from Cuschier A, Szabo Z: *Tissue Approximation in Endoscopic Surgery*, Isis Medical Media, Oxford, UK, 1995, used with permission.)

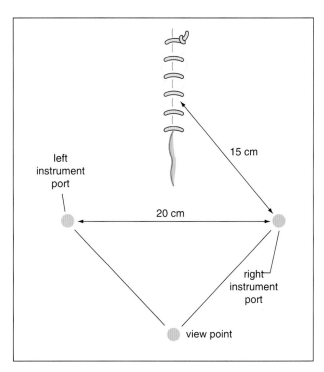

Figure 3.236 A diamond should be formed with the laparoscope, needle holder, assistor, and the suture line to minimize frustration.

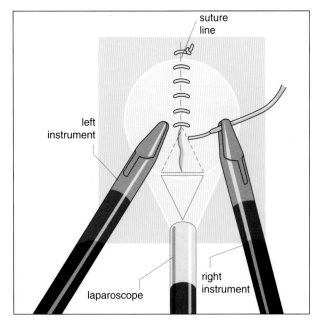

Figure 3.235 The coaxial laparoscopic view enables the physician to see each instrument completely, similar to the view seen at open laparotomy.

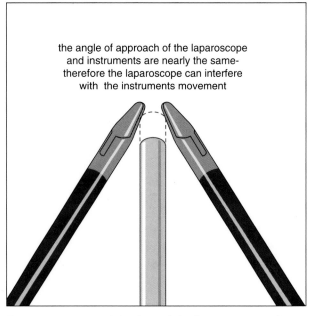

Figure 3.237 A pelvic view of the laparoscope and instruments.

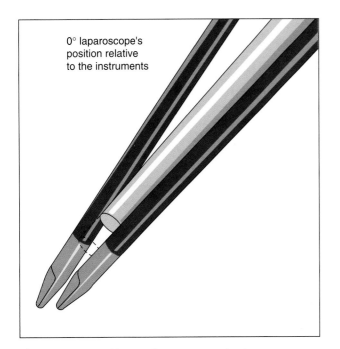

Figure 3.238 With a 0° laparoscope, the instruments will need to be slightly deeper to avoid possible 'crossing of swords'.

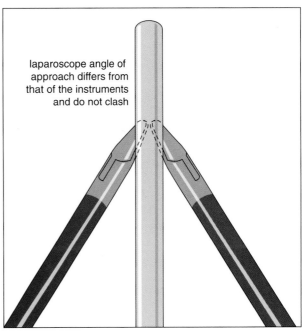

Figure 3.239 If the scope is inserted too deeply, the instruments will clash.

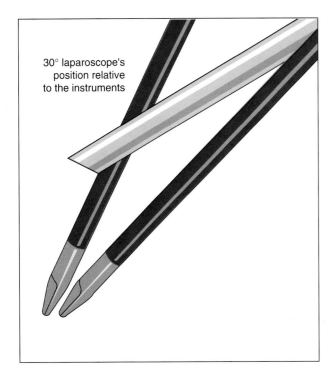

Figure 2.240 To avoid instrument clash, a 30° scope is used to view the instruments from a superior angle.

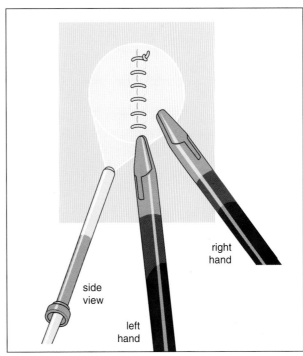

Figure 2.241 Placing the scope from the side may limit full view of the suture site by the needle holder or the tissue grasper.

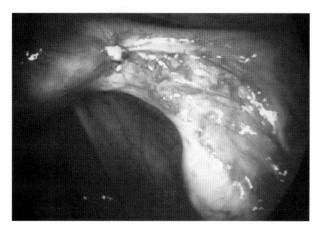

*Figure 3.242 This patient had previously undergone a bipolar cautery tubal ligation. There appeared to be adequate cornual portions of the tube, as well as adequate distal tubes with normal fimbrae.

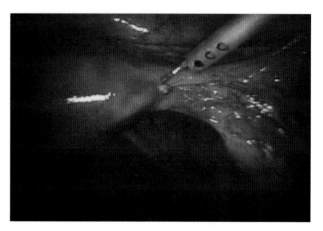

Figure 3.243 The diode laser is used with the conical tipped fiber at 6 watts to mobilize the mid-portions of the tube away from the mesosalpinx. The serosal and muscularis portions of the tube are dissected away from the mucosa using the laser technique. This technique reduces the need for irrigation and cautery, as bleeding is usually minimal.

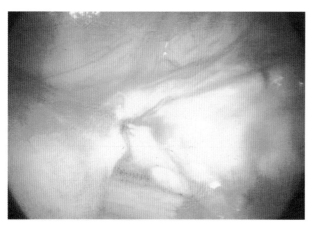

Figure 3.244 Hemostasis is maintained as the tubal stumps are mobilized.

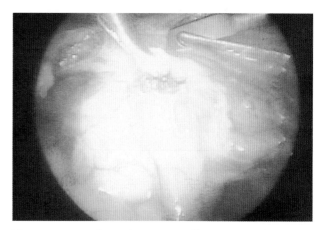

Figure 3.245 The endoscopic guillotine is used to make the final cut across the tubal mucosa. The tubal stump is grasped.

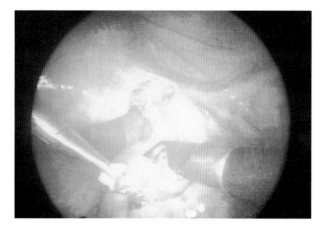

Figure 3.246 The tubal stump is positioned into the guillotine blade.

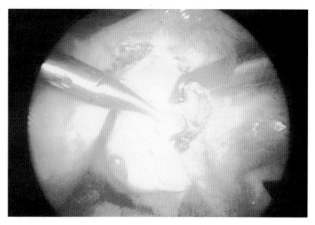

Figure 3.247 The occluded tubal stump is removed after the blade has been extended.

* The quality of Figures 3.242 to 3.255 is due to the technical difficulties in photographing the procedure.

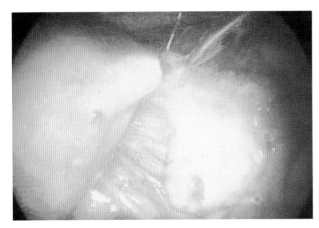

Figure 3.248 The proximal and distal portions of the tube are confirmed patent by hydrotubation and by probing.

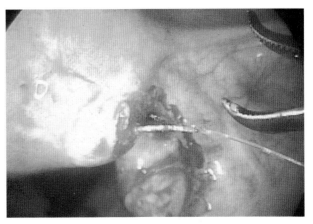

Figure 3.249 Stents, although initially tried, have been eliminated from the standard technique.

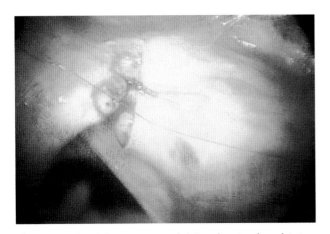

Figure 3.250 A base suture of 4-0 nylon is placed into the mesosalpinx to help align the tube, and reduce tension from the tubal sutures.

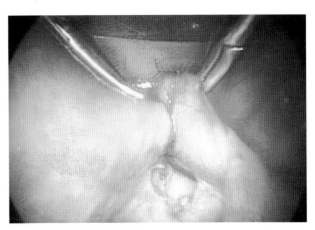

Figure 3.251 Four sutures of 6-0 nylon are placed into each quadrant of the tubal opening, through the serosa, muscularis, and mucosa.

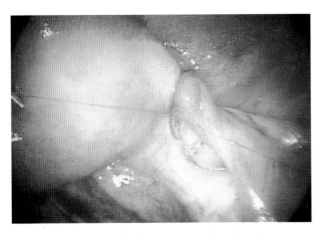

Figure 3.252 The tubal junction is aligned as the suture is cinched down to the tissue.

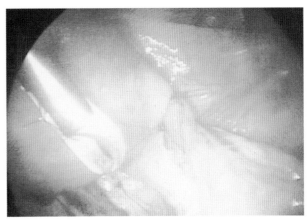

Figure 3.253 The nylon is trimmed.

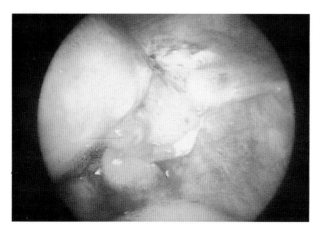

Figure 3.254 Additional sutures are placed.

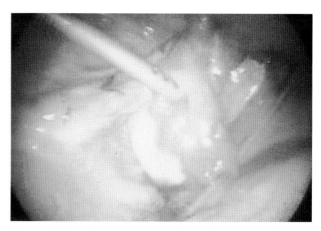

Figure 3.255 Hydrotubation is carried out to confirm patency at the conclusion of the procedure.

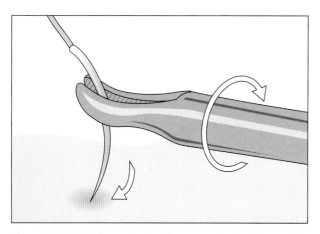

Figure 3.256 When suturing laparoscopically, the needle should be grasped near the hub on the flat portion of the curve. The needle holder should be rotated, prior to placing the needle into the tissue, to be sure that no obstruction will be encountered upon needle placement.

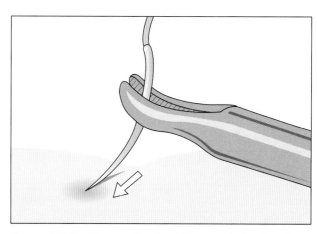

Figure 3.257 The needle should be precisely placed into the tissue.

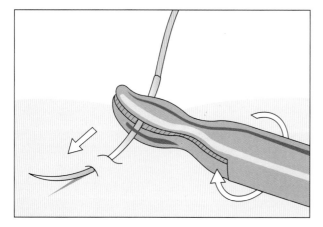

Figure 3.258 A deliberate rotating movement is used to place the needle through the tissue. Sometimes, the tissue is concomitantly brought onto the needle.

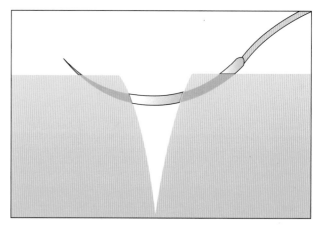

Figure 3.259 This transverse view shows that the needle should contain an equal amount of tissue, at the same depth and width for both sides.

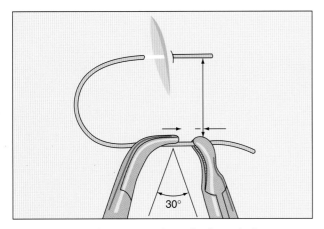

Figure 3.260 The suture is brought through the tissue, and the needle holder regrasps the suture about 6–7 cm from the tissue in preparation for intracorporeal knot tying.

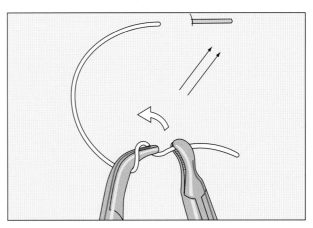

Figure 3.261 The suture is wound around the assistor once.

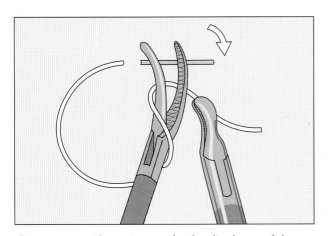

Figure 3.262 The assistor grabs the distal part of the suture.

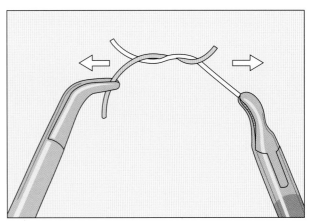

Figure 3.263 The first throw is completed as the knot is brought toward the tissue's suture line.

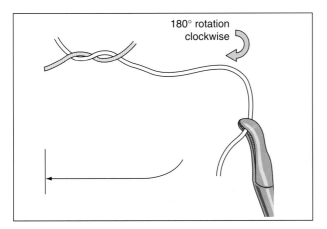

Figure 3.264 The short end of the suture is grasped by the needle holder.

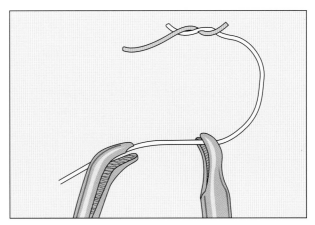

Figure 3.265 The suture from the needle holder is handed to the assistor.

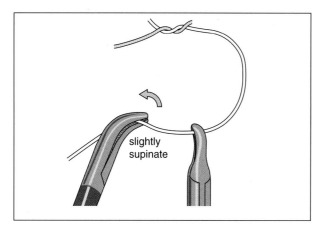

Figure 3.266   The assistor elevates the suture above the needle holder to start to wrap the suture around the needle holder.

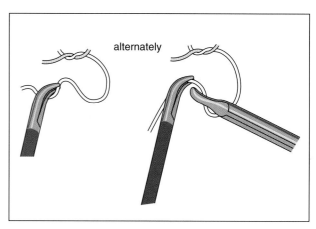

Figure 3.267   The assistor or the needle holder may be primarily used to wrap the suture, but care should be taken to facilitate a square knot by wrapping the suture the same way as the first throw was done.

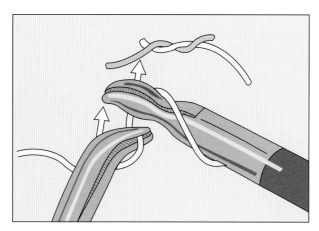

Figure 3.268   Both the assistor and the needle holder need to move in unison toward the short end of the suture near the suture line.

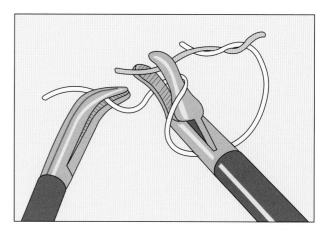

Figure 3.269   The short end of the suture is grasped by the needle holder.

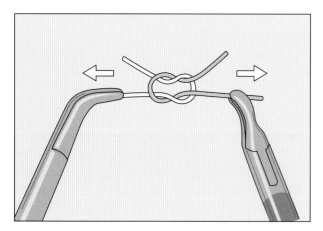

Figure 3.270   A square knot results when the proper technique is used.

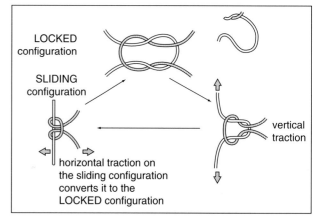

Figure 3.271   One is able to convert the knot to a slip knot to cinch the suture tighter toward the tissue if needed.

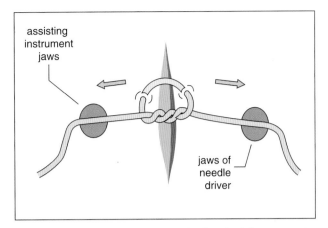

Figure 3.272 When viewed at the level of the suture, it is important to be sure that the instrument jaws are parallel to the suture, when tightening the knot, in order to avoid breaking the suture.

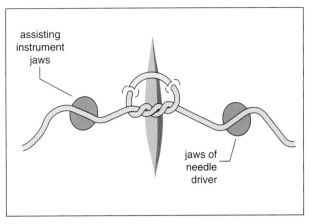

Figure 3.273 This diagram shows an improper technique, which will result in extreme frustration in attempting laparoscopic microsurgical tubal reanastomosis.

Operative hysteroscopy – operating room set-up

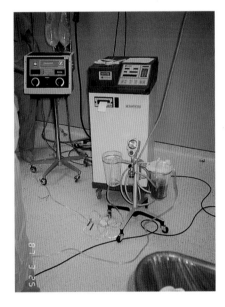

Figure 3.274 The Nd:YAG laser is primarily used for operative hysteroscopy.

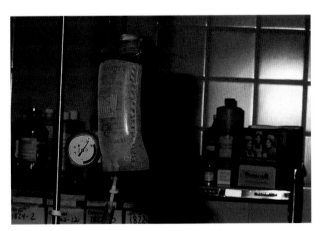

Figure 3.275 Fluid may be infused using a blood infusion pump.

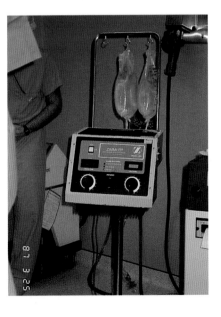

Figure 3.276 Fluid may be infused using a constant-flow infusion pump.

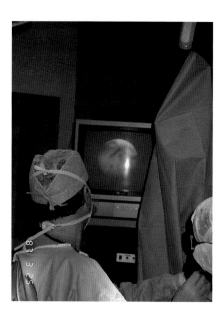

Figure 3.277 The procedure may be viewed on a high-resolution TV monitor by coupling the camera directly to the hysteroscope.

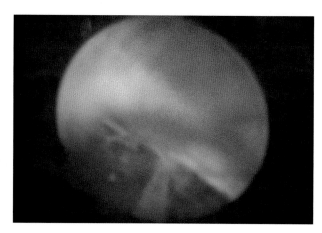

Figure 3.278 The fiber is seen inside the uterus on the monitor. The operating personnel are still cautioned to use protective goggles in case of accidental fiber disruption while the laser is activated.

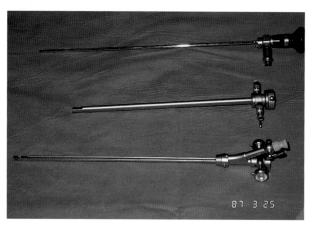

Figure 3.279 The laser hysteroscope with an albarran bridge is displayed.

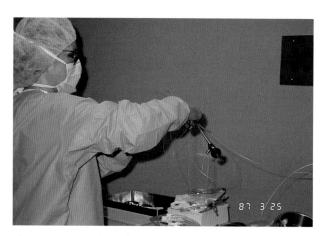

Figure 3.280 The infusion fluid tubing and a laser fiber are brought over the surgical field.

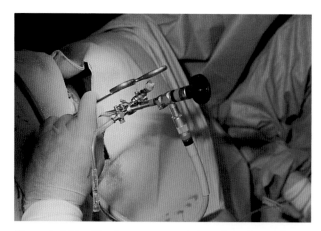

Figure 3.281 The hysteroscope is introduced into the uterine cavity.

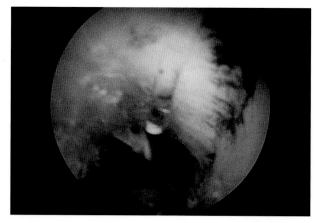

Figure 3.282 The Nd:YAG bare fiber is noted with aiming beam on.

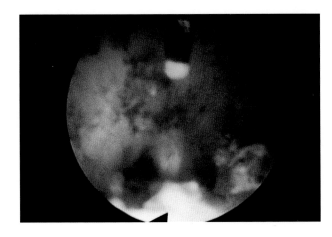

Figure 3.283 Either a contact or non-contact technique may be used with a bare fiber to vaporize the endometrial lining; usually 60–80 watts of power is needed. The endometrium has been atrophied by using Depot Lupron at least one month prior to the procedure; a second injection is usually given on the day of surgery.

Laser metroplasty

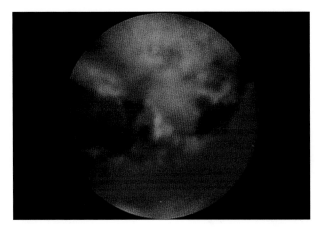

Figure 3.284 Transcervical hysteroscopic metroplasty may be performed using either a bare fiber or contact drawn fiber with the Nd:YAG laser. The sapphire tips should *not* be used with gas cooling as fatal air embolus may occur.

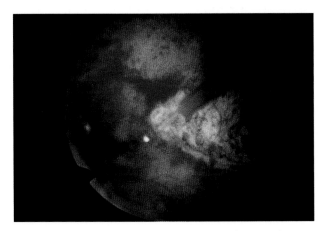

Figure 3.285 The septum is approached from each cornua with the contact YAG fiber using 12 watts of power.

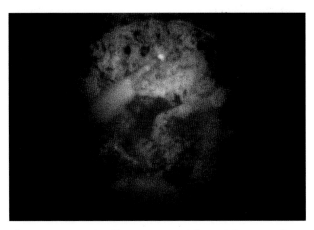

Figure 3.286 The fiber is swept right to left across the septum. Minimal bleeding is usually encountered.

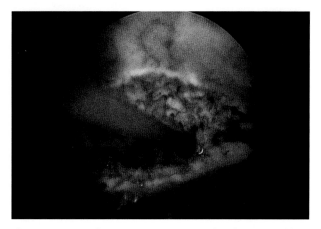

Figure 3.287 The septum is continued to be incised by the laser fiber.

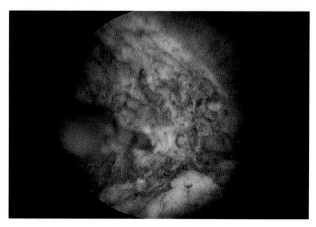

Figure 3.288 The metroplasty is completed.

Sub-mucous myomectomy – laser and electrocautery

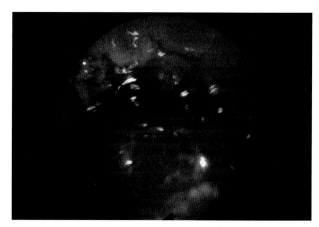

Figure 3.289 Note the CO_2 hysteroscopic view of a sub-mucous myoma. CO_2 as a distending medium should be used for diagnostic purposes only.

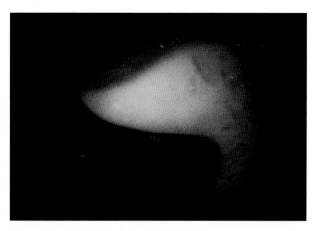

Figure 3.290 Note the view of a sub-mucous myoma using Ringers lactate as the distending medium.

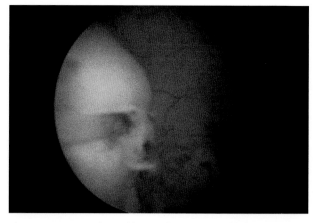

Figure 3.291 A bare fiber Nd:YAG laser fiber is used at 60 watts of power to vaporize the fibroid.

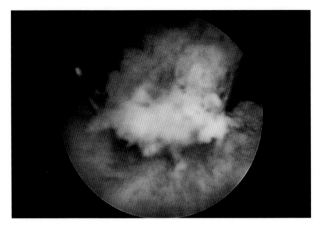

Figure 3.292 An electrocautery loop to excise the fibroid works more rapidly.

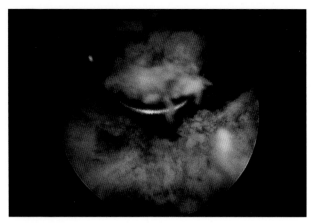

Figure 3.293 Sorbitol or glycine is used to allow the electro-energy to work. The resectoscope is brought toward the operator when the Bovie is activated; the loop should be viewed at all times prior to activating the electrical energy.

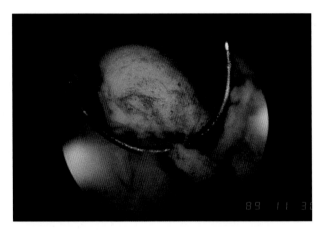

Figure 3.294 Note the absence of bleeding.

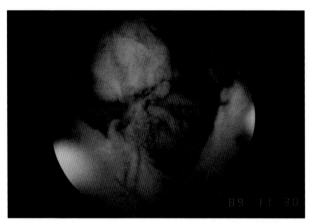

Figure 3.295 A furrow in the myoma is made by the electrical loops.

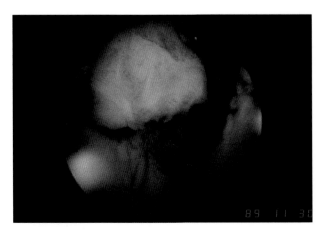

Figure 3.296 A myoma is excised.

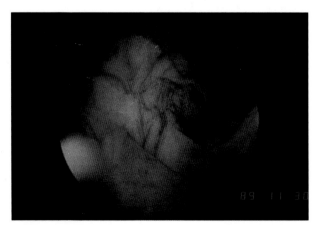

Figure 3.297 Note the furrow which remains after excision of a myoma.

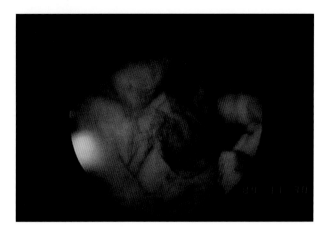

Figure 3.298   The myoma usually cannot be removed entirely as it is resected to the level of the uterine cavity.

Endometrial ablation

Laser technique

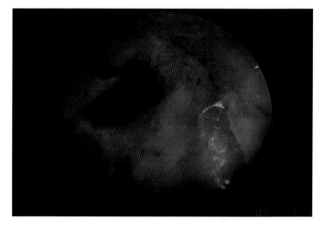

Figure 3.299   Endometrial ablation may be accomplished using a bare fiber Nd:YAG laser at 60–80 watts. Again the endometrium is prepared by using Depot Lupron pre-operatively.

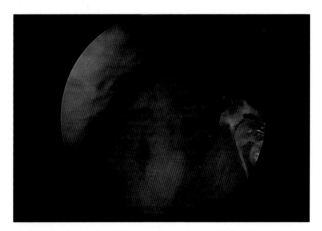

Figure 3.300   The fiber is drawn toward the operator starting at the most distal point using a contact or non-contact technique.

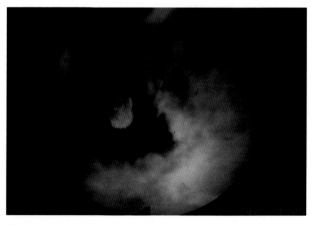

Figure 3.301   This patient required a repeat endometrial ablation six months later for a small amount of active endometrium which remained near the lower uterine segment.

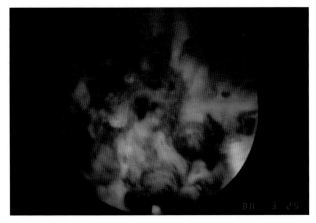

Figure 3.302 This is what the endometrium should look like at the conclusion of the endometrial ablation.

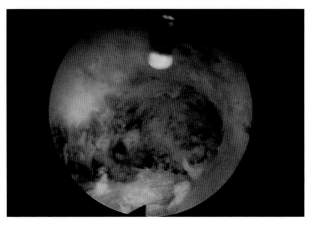

Figure 3.303 This is an endometrial ablation with the non-contact technique using a bare Nd:YAG fiber.

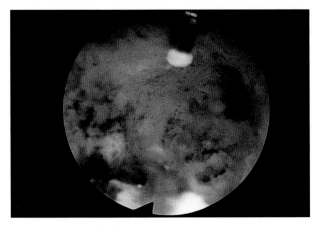

Figure 3.304 Blanching is noted with some carbonization as the energy is applied.

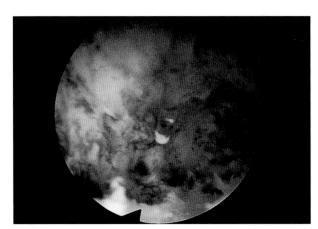

Figure 3.305 Blanching is nearly completed.

Rollerball technique

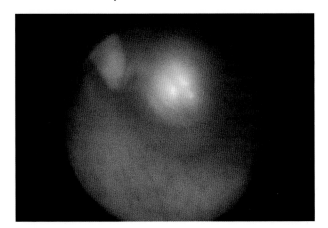

Figure 3.306 The electrocautery rollerball works more rapidly. The power setting is usually 40 watts cutting. Upon distending the uterus, some blood may be encountered which may initially obscure the field.

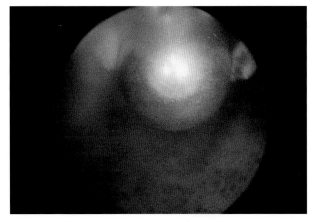

Figure 3.307 The continuous flow hysteroscope should be used to help clear the field of blood prior to starting the endometrial ablation.

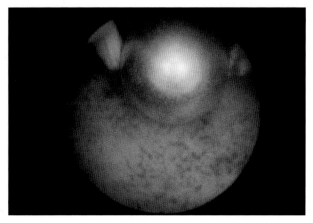

Figure 3.308 The rollerball is brought toward the operator again keeping contact with the tissue and viewing the rollerball at all times.

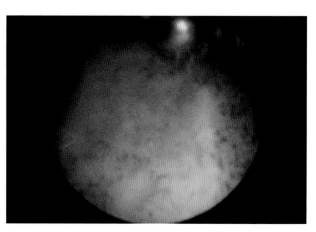

Figure 3.309 Blanching is noted from the electrocautery effect of the rollerball.

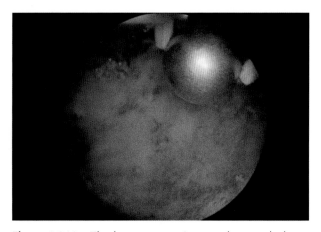

Figure 3.310 The hysteroscope is rotated to reach the anterior and lateral walls of the endometrial cavity.

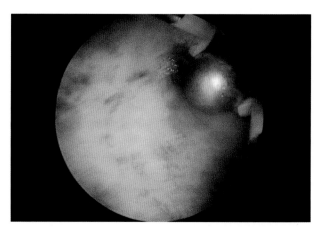

Figure 3.311 The cornua is usually the most difficult spot to reach. Care must be taken to avoid prolonged exposure of the electricity at this point which is the thinnest area of the uterus.

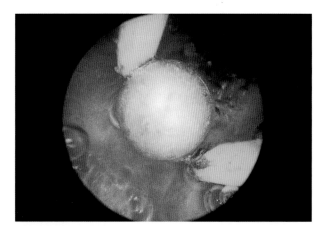

Figure 3.312 Bubbles may be encountered as the endometrial ablation continues. These should be of minimal concern unless the view becomes obscured.

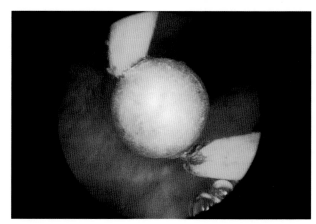

Figure 3.313 The ablation is continued as the hysteroscope with the rollerball is rotated.

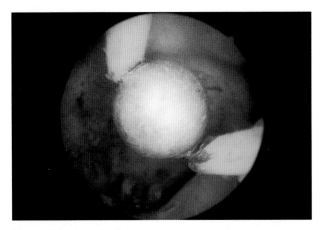

Figure 3.314 All of the walls are treated.

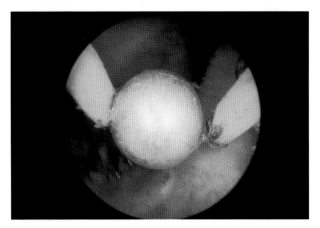

Figure 3.315 The endometrial ablation is nearly completed. Usually the procedure may be accomplished in 30–60 minutes, depending on the size of the uterine cavity and the skill of the operator and operating room personnel.

ThermaChoice™ uterine balloon therapy

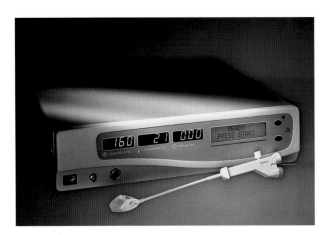

Figure 3.316 ThermaChoice™ uterine balloon therapy is devised to ablate the endometrial lining in premenopausal women, who have completed their families, with menorrhagia due to benign causes. About 85% of patients report reduced post-operative menstrual bleeding to normal or less following this 8 minute outpatient procedure. The patient selection criteria include: documented menorrhagia, normal Pap smear and endometrial sampling, premenopausal patients who have completed childbearing, a uterine cavity of 6–10 cm, and failed or contraindicated medical therapy. The thermal balloon conforms to the intra-uterine configuration in order to maximize contact with the endometrium. ThermaChoice™ is contraindicated in patients with a latex allergy, those who wish to become pregnant, those with endometrial hyperplasia or malignancy, those with active pelvic or urinary tract infection, or those with a significant uterine incision (transmural myomectomy or classical C-section).

Thermal endometrial ablation with ThermaChoice™ How it works:

- Catheter with heater at tip enclosed in a balloon
- Balloon catheter inserted through cervix into uterus

- Balloon filled with sterile fluid
- Expands to fit size and shape of uterus

- Fluid in balloon is heated during 8 min treatment cycle
- Uterine lining is destroyed
- Cather is removed and discarded

Figure 3.317 The balloon device is inserted transcervically, similar to an intra-uterine device, filled with sterile fluid until the intra-uterine pressure reaches 160–180 mmHg. The heating element raises the balloon temperature to 187°F (86°C), and maintains it for 8 minutes. When the controller signals that treatment is complete, the balloon is deflated, the catheter removed, and then discarded. The patient is released home after recovering from the outpatient general anesthesia.

Tubal cannulation

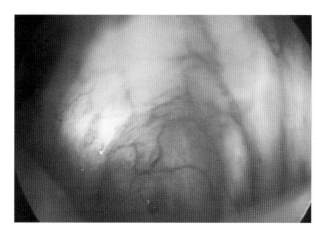

Figure 3.318 To evaluate cornual occlusion, a hysteroscopic view of the tubal ostia is required using either a fluid or gas (CO_2) medium.

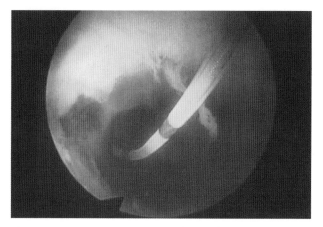

Figure 3.319 Using a Novy catheter, the ostia is probed for an opening. If a true occlusion is confirmed, either IVF or microlaser cornual resection/reanastomosis would be advised.

BIBLIOGRAPHY

Amso NN, Stabinsky SA, McFaul P, et al: Uterine thermal balloon therapy for the treatment of menorrhagia: the first 300 patients from a multi-centre study. *Br J Obstet Gynaecol* **105**:507–23, 1998.

Baggish MS, Barbot J, Valle RF: *Diagnostic and Operative Hysteroscopy, a Text and Atlas.* Chicago, Year Book Medical Publishers, 1989.

Baggish M, Diamond M: Hysteroscopy overview: instrumentation methodology/complications. In: *Contemporary Endoscopy, Syllabus for 24th Annual Post-graduate Course.* Birmingham, American Fertility Society, 1991.

Bateman B, Kolp L, Mills S: Endoscopic versus laparotomy management of endometriomas. *Fertil Steril* **62**:690–5, 1994.

Brooks PG: Operative hysteroscopy. In Pitkin RM, Scott JR (eds): *Clinical Obstetrics and Gynecology* Philadelphia, J.B. Lippincott, Vol. 35, 1992.

Carter J: Laparoscopic treatment of chronic pelvic pain in 100 adult women. *J Am Assoc Gynecol Laparosc* **2**:255–62, 1995.

Cohen M, Evantash E: Laparoscopic sterilization reversal. *Infertil Reprod Med Clin North Am* **8**:443–7, 1997.

Cushieri A, Szabo Z: *Tissue Approximation in Endoscopic Surgery.* Oxford, U.K., Isis Medical Media, 1995.

Dawood M, Ramos J, Khan-Dawood F: Depot leuprolide acetate versus danazol for treatment of pelvic endometriosis: changes in vertebral bone mass and serum estradiol and calcitonin. *Fertil Steril* **63**:1177–83, 1995.

Diamond MP: Pelviscopy. In Pitkin RM, Scott JR (eds): *Clinical Obstetrics and Gynecology.* Philadelphia, J.B. Lippincott, Vol. 34, 1992.

Falcone T, Goldberg J, Miller K: Endometriosis: medical and surgical intervention. *Curr Opin Obstet Gynecol* **8**:178–83, 1996.

Gjonnaess H: Late endocrine effects of ovarian electrocautery in women with polycystic ovary syndrome. *Fertil Steril* **69**:697–701, 1998.

Gomel V: From microsurgery to laparoscopic surgery: a progress. *Fertil Steril* **63**:464–8, 1995.

Johns A: Laparoscopy overview: instrumentation/ methodology/complications. In: *Contemporary Endoscopy, Syllabus for 24th Annual Post-graduate Course.* Birmingham, American Fertility Society, 1991.

Lu P, Ory S: Endometriosis: current management. *Mayo Clin Proc* **70**:453–63, 1995.

Marcoux S, Maheux R, Berube S, et al: Laparoscopic surgery in infertile women with minimal or mild endometriosis. *N Engl J Med* **337**:217–22, 1997.

Margossian H, Garcia-Ruiz A, Falcone T, et al: Robotically assisted laparoscopic microsurgical uterine horn anastomosis. *Fertil Steril* **70**:530–4, 1998.

McLaughlin DS (ed.): *Lasers in Gynecology*. Philadelphia, J.B. Lippincott, 1991.

McLucas B, Morales AJ, Murphy AA: Endoscopic surgery in gynecology. In: *Current Problems in Obstetrics, Gynecology, and Fertility*. St. Louis, Mosby-Year Book, Vol. 15, 1992.

Meyer WR, Walsh BW, Grainger DA, et al: Thermal balloon and rollerball ablation to treat menorrhagia: a multicenter comparison. *Obstet Gynecol* **92**:98–103, 1998.

Nieuwkerk P, Hagenius P, Ankum W, et al: Systemic methotrexate therapy versus laparoscopic salpingostomy in patients with tubal pregnancy. Part 1. Impact on patients' health-related quality of life. *Fertil Steril* **70**:511–17, 1998.

Olive D, Schwartz L: Medical progress: endometriosis. *N Engl J Med* **328**:1759–69, 1993.

Orwoll E, Yuzpe A, Burry K, et al: Nafarelin therapy in endometriosis: long-term effects on bone mineral density. *Am J Obstet Gynecol* **171**:1221–5, 1994.

Semm K, Friedrich ER (eds): *Operative Manual for Endoscopic Abdominal Surgery*. Chicago, Year Book Medical Publishers, 1987.

Siegler AM, Lindemann HJ: *Hysteroscopy Principles and Practice*. Philadelphia, J.B. Lippincott, 1984.

Summit R, Stovall T, Steege J, et al: A multicenter randomized comparison of laparoscopically assisted vaginal hysterectomy and abdominal hysterectomy in abdominal hysterectomy candidates. *Obstet Gynecol* **92**:321–6, 1998.

Sutton C, Ewen S, Whitelaw N, Haines P: Prospective, randomized, double-blind, controlled trial of laser laparoscopy in the treatment of pelvic pain associated with minimal, mild, and moderate endometriosis. *Fertil Steril* **62**:696–700, 1994.

Tulandi T, Bugnah M: Operative laparoscopy: surgical modalities. *Fertil Steril* **63**:237–45, 1995.

Yao M, Tulandi T: Current status of surgical and nonsurgical management of ectopic pregnancy. *Fertil Steril* **67**:421–33, 1997.

Yoon, T, Sung H, Cha S, et al: Fertility outcome after laparoscopic microsurgical tubal anastomosis. *Fertil Steril* **67**:18–22, 1997.

4 Microlaser surgery

Intra-abdominal gynecological laser surgery was initially introduced by Bellina in 1974, and subsequently popularized by Baggish, Chong, Daniell, Diamond, Feste, McLaughlin, Martin, and other investigators during the following two decades. The carbon dioxide laser is primarily used for open abdominal gynecological procedures. The CO_2 laser's articulating arm may be attached to a hand piece (Fig. 4.1). By attaching the laser to a microslad (Figs 4.2 and 4.3), in conjunction with an operating microscope (Figs 4.4 and 4.5), the laser microsurgeon becomes able to guide the infrared light energy to the appropriate tissue impact site by a joystick (Fig. 4.6). The evolution of microlaser surgery enhanced the CO_2 laser's ability to destroy pathology more precisely. By reflecting the beam off a molybdenum mirror (Figs 4.7 and 4.8), the laser energy could be applied to previously inaccessible areas. Ebonized laser instruments (Figs 4.9–4.15) were developed to prevent accidental reflection of the laser's energy to vital intra-abdominal structures. Angled quartz rods (Figs 4.10–4.19) were designed, which provide an excellent absorptive backstop for laser energy to facilitate the vaporization of adhesions coapting normal tissue. A smoke evacuation system (Fig. 4.20) is needed on the surgical field to properly remove the toxic laser smoke (Fig. 4.21). The development of specific instrumentation has enhanced the CO_2 laser's inherent properties of precision, hemostasis, and the ability to reach previously inaccessible sites. These unique laser properties have been successfully applied to gynecology in order to enhance or preserve reproductive potential (Table 4.1).

An organized approach to microlaser surgery includes the use of a dual-headed operating microscope (Fig. 4.22) with a 300 mm objective lens, coupled to the laser via a microslad using a 300 mm laser lens. No sterile drape is used, as the laser's energy would melt the plastic at the exit port. A sterile angiocath cover or the tip of a Robinson urinary catheter is used to cover the joystick (Fig. 4.23). Shortened, ebonized stainless steel instruments are used in conjunction with angled quartz rods and

Table 4.1 Indications for microlaser surgery

- Vaporization of adhesions
- Vaporization of endometriosis
- Excision of ovarian cysts
- Ovarian wedge resection for polycystic ovaries
- Fimbrioplasty
- Neosalpingostomy
- Tubal reanastomosis
- Removing cornual polyps
- Myomectomy
- Metroplasty
- Ectopic pregnancy

molybdenum mirrors. Moistened non-woven laparotomy sponges are used to insulate vital intra-abdominal structures from inadvertent laser energy. Varying power densities are used for different intra-abdominal applications (Table 4.2). High power densities ($>18,000$ W/cm^2) are achieved using 35 watts of superpulse with a 0.2 mm spot. Lower power densities are achieved by reducing the wattage and/or defocusing the spot (e.g. 10 watts non-superpulse, 1 mm spot). It is important to reduce the thermal imprint left on the remaining tissue by using rapid joystick movements with the highest power density which is appropriate to achieve the desired result.

Adhesion reformation may be minimized by using a gentle microsurgical technique with an effort made to use instruments and suture to minimize bleeding and subsequent adhesion reformation (e.g. laser and siliconized braided nylon sutures). A recent report by Diamond and the Sepracoat Adhesion Study Group concluded that HAL-C solution (Sepracoat) was significantly safe and effective in reducing the incidence, extent, and severity of de novo adhesion formation following gynecological laparotomy.

Table 4.2 Recommended power densities

High (35 watts superpulse, finely focused spot)
- Excising adhesions
- Excising ovarian cysts
- Ovarian wedge resection
- Myomectomy
- Metroplasty
- Fimbrioplasty—incising adhesive collar
- Neosalpingostomy—stellate incision
- Tubal reanastomosis—excising scar (except tubal mucosa)

Low (10 watts non-superpulse, defocused beam)
- Vaporizing adhesions
- Vaporizing endometriosis—directly and indirectly
- Vaporizing small fibroids
- 'Brushing' surface-ovarian adhesions
- Bruhat maneuver—everting distal tubal serosa for fimbrioplasty or neosalpingostomy

Additionally, the gynecologist should consider colorectal involvement of endometriosis based on the symptoms of pelvic and rectal pain. When the cul-de-sac is significantly involved, a team approach coordinating a general surgeon with a pre-operative bowel preparation will enable complete treatment of extensive disease, which may include bowel resection. Although often technically difficult, these complete operations can accomplish good symptomatic relief, acceptable pregnancy rates, and low morbidity.

Also, Tjaden et al reported their prospective study used to evaluate the efficacy of presacral neurectomy for central pain relief. They concluded that it is highly effective for refractory dysmenorrhea, and that presumed failure of the procedure was inappropriate selection of surgical candidates or incomplete resection of the presacral nerve plexus.

The subsequent figures (Figs 4.24–4.166) will more clearly illustrate the intra-abdominal applications of the CO_2 laser in fertility promoting/preserving procedures.

Operating room set-up

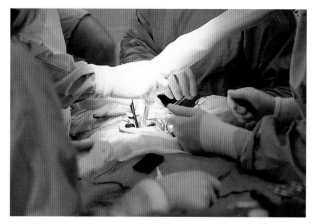

Figure 4.1 Laser hand piece attached to the articulating arm gives a high power density due to the short focal length of the laser lens (125 mm). This set-up is useful for excising large tumors such as large myomas.

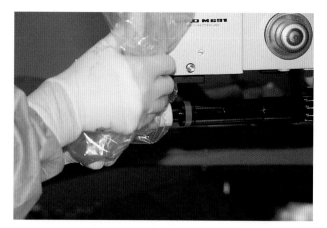

Figure 4.2 A CO_2 laser attached to a Sharplan microslad which has varying spot size and a Wilde microscope.

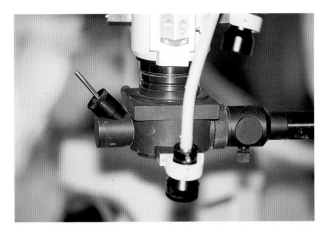

Figure 4.3 A CO_2 laser attached to a Sharplan microslad and a Zeiss microscope. The microslad connects the articulating arm of the CO_2 laser to the base of the operating microscope. The laser lens (300 mm) needs to match the microscope objective (300 mm) in order to minimize the spot, thus maximizing the power density.

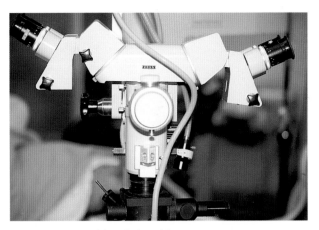

Figure 4.4 Dual-headed Wilde microscope.

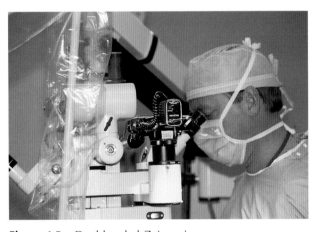

Figure 4.5 Dual-headed Zeiss microscope.

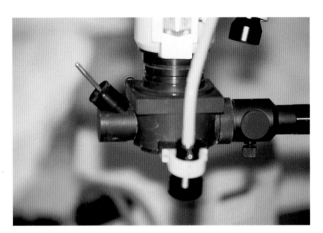

Figure 4.6 Non-sterile joystick of microslad to direct CO_2 laser beam.

Laser instruments

Figure 4.7 The molybdenum mirror is used intra-operatively in order to visualize pathology on the under surfaces of the pelvic organs. The laser beam can be fired directly into the mirror and reflected to the pathologic site. This is opposite to the dentist's technique in which he/she uses the mirror to visualize the pathology and operates directly on the pathologic site.

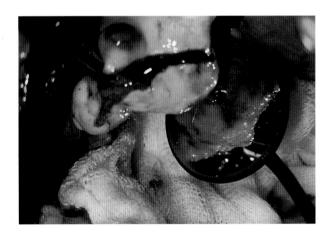

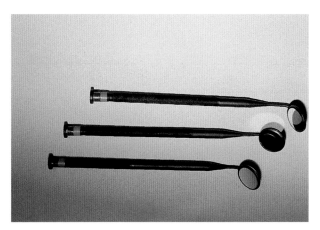

Figure 4.8 The molybdenum mirrors are angled at 30°, 60°, and 90° in order to enable the laser to reflect optimally and strike the surgical site at a perpendicular angle.

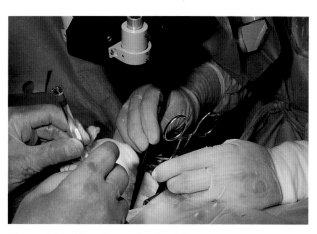

Figure 4.9 Microlaser ebonized instruments were specially adapted and created to facilitate microlaser surgery.

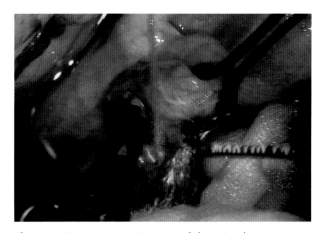

Figure 4.10 Microscopic view of the microlaser instruments of Fig. 4.9.

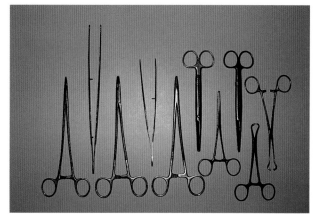

Figure 4.11 The laser set consists of tissue pick-ups, needle holders, hemostats, Babcock clamps, towel clamps, and scissors. They are a maximum of eight inches in length to avoid contaminating the instrument on the non-sterile microslad during microlaser surgery.

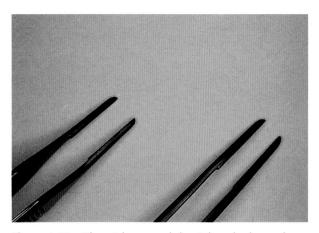

Figure 4.12 The pick-ups and the Babcock clamps have carbide inserts which atraumatically hold the tissue.

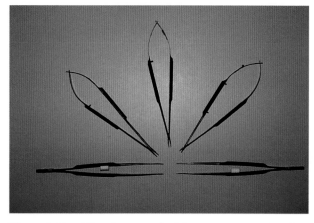

Figure 4.13 Microlaser surgical instruments consist of straight and angled needle holders, tissue forceps, and microscissors to facilitate microsurgery.

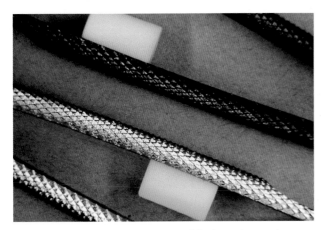

Figure 4.14 The instruments are blackened to reduce the reflectivity of the CO_2 laser which may inadvertently strike vital intra-abdominal structures. Ebonized instruments also have less glare, which enables the surgeon to complete his/her surgery with less eye fatigue.

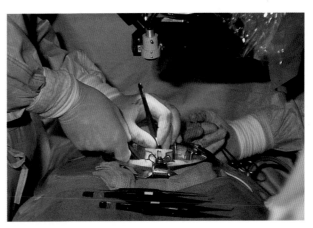

Figure 4.15 Note the proximity of the eight-inch laser instruments to the non-sterile microslad.

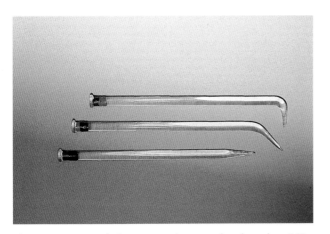

Figure 4.16 Angled quartz rods were developed at 60°, 90°, and 180° to act as a backstop and absorb the laser's energy.

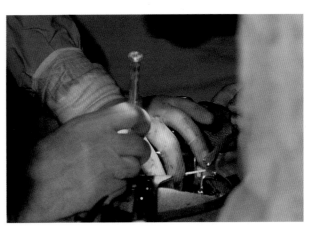

Figure 4.17 The quartz rods have a maximum length of eight inches to avoid contamination from the non-sterile microslad during laser surgery.

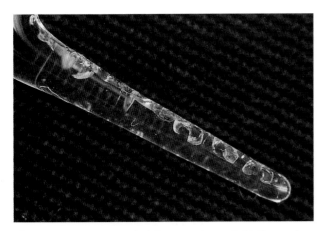

Figure 4.18 An annealed Pyrex rod was initially used, however, due to internal crystal disruption (laser crazing), the rods fractured after a short time of use.

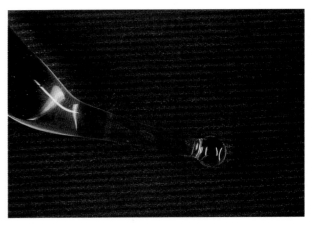

Figure 4.19 Quartz is able to withstand the laser impact in a much more durable fashion than Pyrex. Laser crazing is reduced, although the rod should be discarded when significant internal crystal disruption becomes apparent.

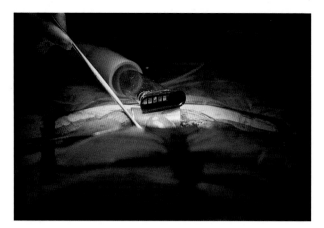

Figure 4.20 The large suction tubing from the smoke evacuator is attached to the plastic drape overlying the patient's abdomen. The closer the suction tip can be placed to the production of surgical smoke, the less likely the operating staff will inhale the toxic substance.

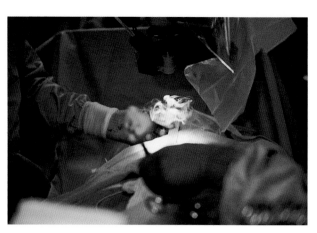

Figure 4.21 Note the puff of smoke produced by the CO_2 laser without the aid of the suction apparatus.

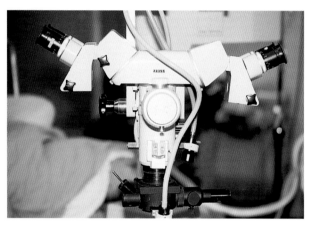

Figure 4.22 The dual-headed microscope allows the operating surgeon, as well as the assistant, to visualize the pelvic structures with a magnified view.

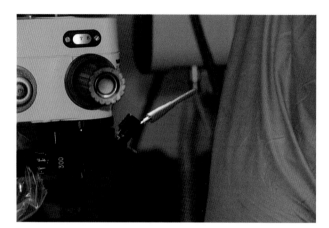

Figure 4.23 Sterile tip of the Robinson catheter used to cover the joystick.

Endometriosis

Direct vaporization

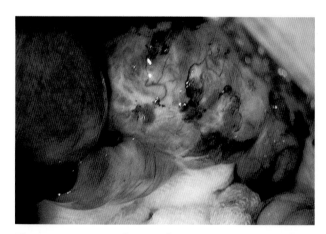

Figure 4.24 Using the CO_2 laser at 10–15 watts with a defocused beam, the joystick should be moved circumferentially with the helium–neon (He–Ne) aiming beam initially over the endometrial implant.

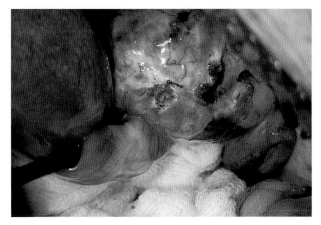

Figure 4.25 The foot pedal, when depressed, activates the CO_2 laser and vaporizes the endometriosis, superficially, to the normal ovarian tissue.

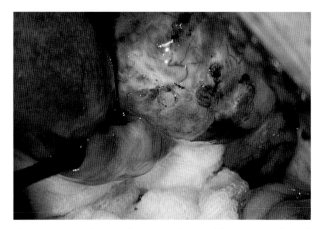

Figure 4.26 The implants are thoroughly vaporized until the normal tissue is seen.

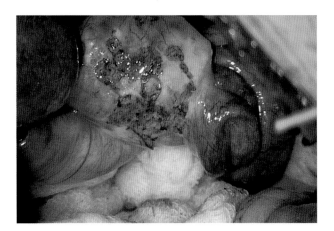

Figure 4.27 The small amount of char can be removed using heparinized Ringers lactate through a small angiocath attached to a syringe.

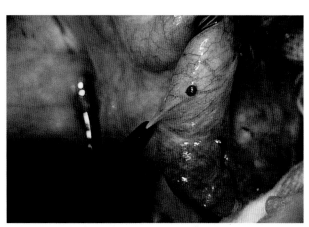

Figure 4.28 Endometriosis on the fallopian tube may be similarly vaporized directly by defocusing the beam using 10 watts of power.

Indirect vaporization

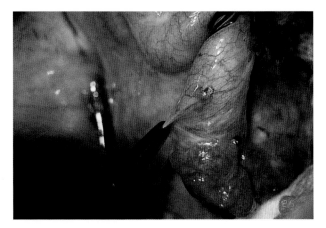

Figure 4.29 It is important to circumferentially ply the He–Ne beam over the site prior to activating the laser.

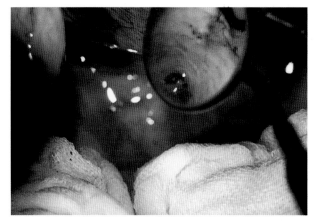

Figure 4.30 The endometriosis is visualized in the molybdenum mirror on the under surface of the pelvic organs.

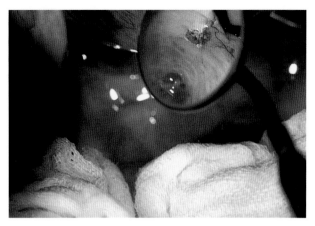

Figure 4.31 Using 10 watts with the defocused beam, the He–Ne beam is circumferentially moved prior to activating the laser. Again note that the surgical procedure is done directly into the mirror so that the beam may be reflected to the pathologic site.

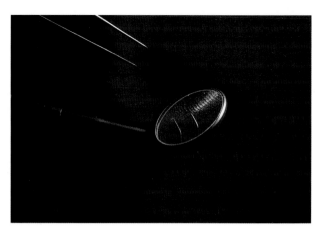

Figure 4.32 This is opposite to how the dentist would directly treat the pathology while visualizing the site in the mirror.

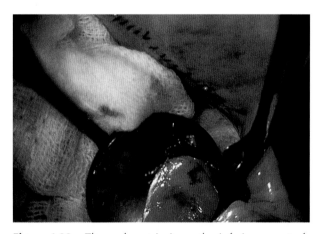

Figure 4.33 The endometriosis on the inferior aspect of the right ovary is visualized in the molybdenum mirror. Moistened non-woven laparotomy sponges are placed in the cul-de-sac in order to avoid accidental injury to the rectum and other vital structures.

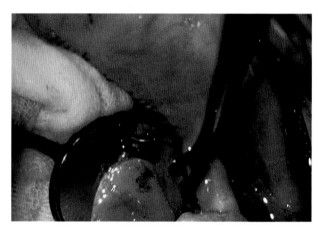

Figure 4.34 The CO_2 laser beam is activated by depressing the foot switch and the endometriosis is vaporized.

Microlaser excision of ovarian endometriomas

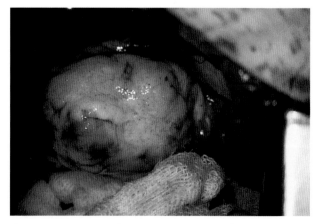

Figure 4.35 An endometrioma deep in the ovary is visualized at the time of laparotomy.

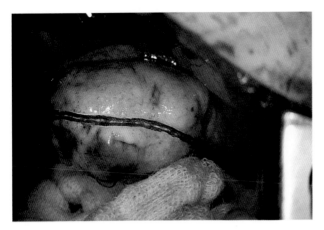

Figure 4.36 Using a finely focused beam (0.2 mm spot) with continuous 35 watts superpulse, an elliptical incision is made on the inferior aspect of the ovary.

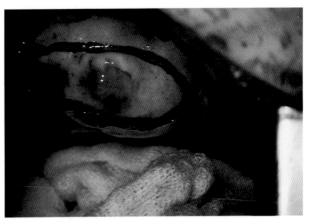

Figure 4.37 The incision is continued until the ellipse is completed.

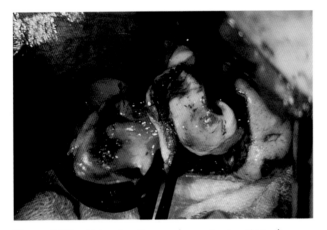

Figure 4.38 Using traction and counter-traction, the laser continues by reflecting the beam into the mirror to strike the surgical site perpendicularly.

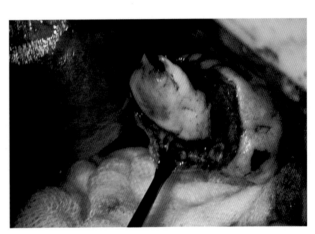

Figure 4.39 The endometrioma is unroofed using laser dissection.

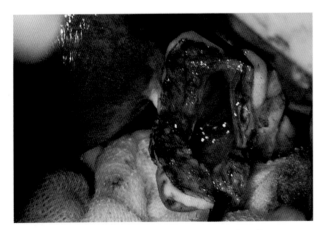

Figure 4.40 The endometrial cyst is visualized. Note the absence of bleeding on the non-woven laparotomy sponges.

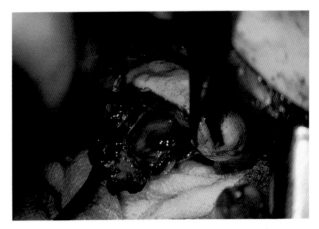

Figure 4.41 With traction and counter-traction the cyst wall is dissected by blunt and laser dissections.

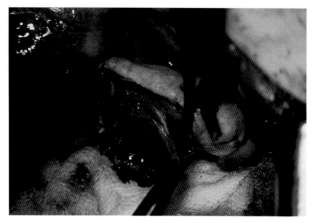

Figure 4.42 Note the hemostasis; usually the cyst wall may be peeled from the remaining normal ovary until the base is reached.

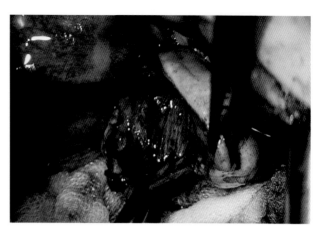

Figure 4.43 Blunt dissection is often the easiest way to remove the cyst.

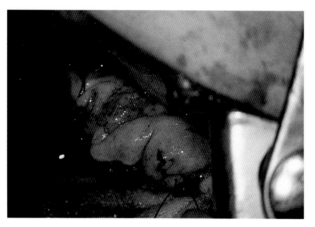

Figure 4.44 The ovary is closed with two deep layers of continuous 4-0 Surgilon.

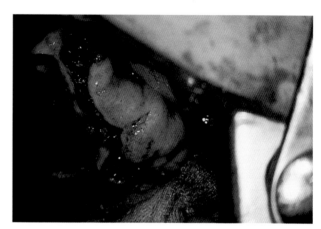

Figure 4.45 Closing of the ovary continues until the cortical layers are in close approximation.

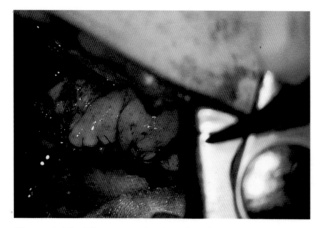

Figure 4.46 The cortex is closed with continuous 4-0 or 6-0 Surgilon depending on the thickness of the cortex and the amount of bleeding.

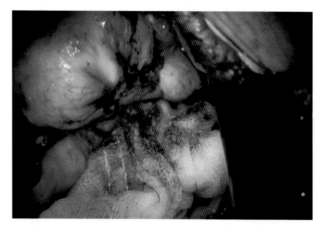

Figure 4.47 Another endometrioma is visualized through the operating microscope with a moistened laparotomy sponge in place.

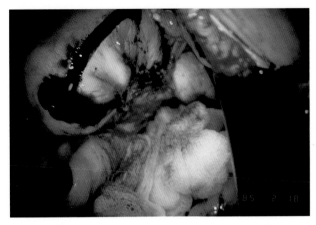

Figure 4.48 Continuous 35 watts superpulse with a 0.2 mm spot is used to make an ellipse directly over the endometrioma.

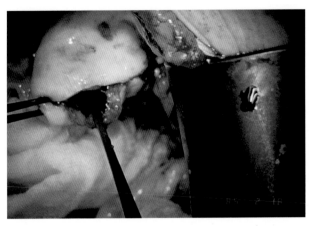

Figure 4.49 Traction and counter-traction are used with carbide-tipped micro-Allis clamps to firmly grasp the tissue without traumatizing it.

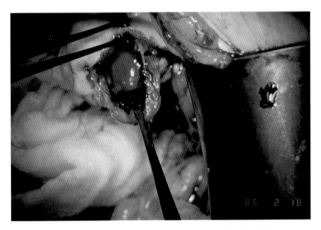

Figure 4.50 The endometrioma is unroofed and drained.

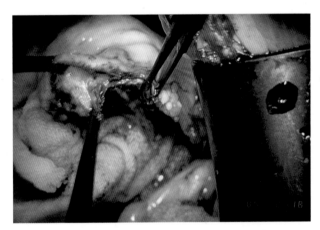

Figure 4.51 The laser is activated to continue the incision until the cyst wall has been completely removed. On occasion part of the cyst remains deep; it may be vaporized entirely by using a circumferential motion of the joystick in a slightly defocused mode.

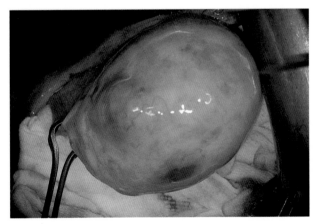

Figure 4.52 Another endometrioma is noted with laparotomy sponges in place. It is sometimes difficult to discern what is normal ovarian tissue versus what is the endometrioma.

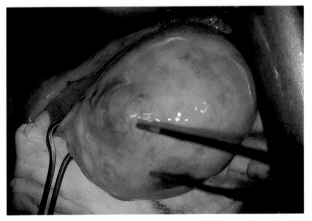

Figure 4.53 The tissue is grasped with the carbide-tipped tissue forceps.

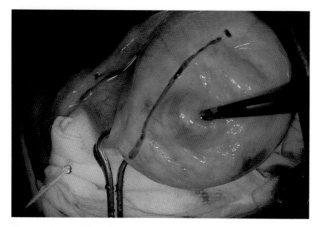

Figure 4.54 The laser incision is made.

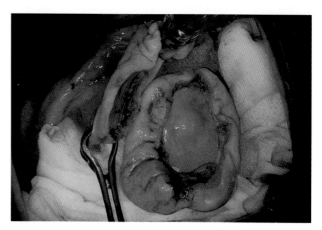

Figure 4.55 The cyst is drained, the endometrioma unroofed, and the base is vaporized.

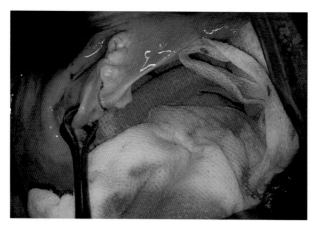

Figure 4.56 Note how the cyst has collapsed completely.

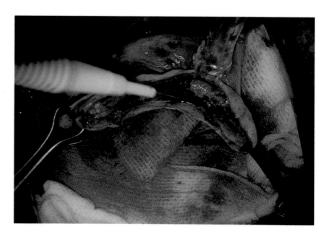

Figure 4.57 Micro-cautery is used to control hemostasis prior to suturing.

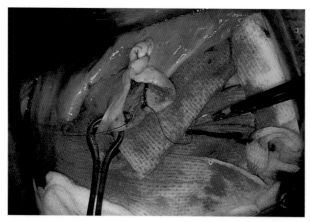

Figure 4.58 Deep sutures of 4-0 Surgilon are placed to approximate the ovary.

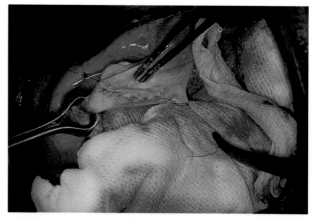

Figure 4.59 Continuous 6-0 Surgilon is used to approximate the cortex.

Bilateral ovarian wedge resection for polycystic ovaries

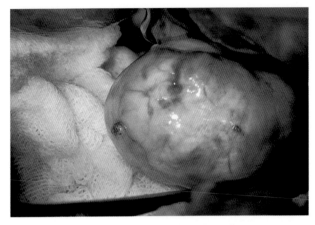

Figure 4.60 This patient had Clomid- and FSH-resistant polycystic ovaries prior to gamete intrafallopian transfer.

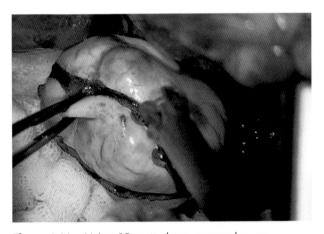

Figure 4.61 Using 35 watts laser superpulse, an elliptical incision is made directly on the inferior lateral aspect of the ovary.

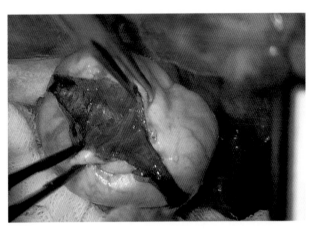

Figure 4.62 Using traction and counter-traction the polycystic ovarian wedge is developed.

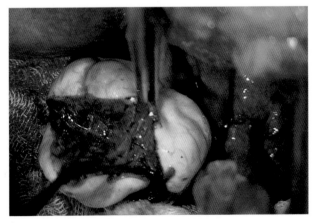

Figure 4.63 The wedge is completely excised with cautery used for hemostasis.

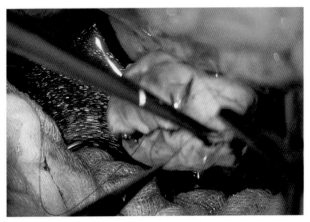

Figure 4.64 Two layers of deep continuous 4-0 Surgilon are used to re-approximate the ovary.

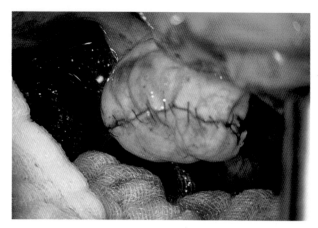

Figure 4.65 Continuous 6-0 Surgilon is used to approximate the cortex entirely. It is important to assure hemostasis in order to reduce the possibility of adhesion reformation post-operatively.

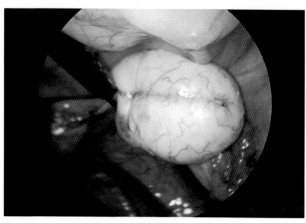

Figure 4.66 Note the excellent healing of the ovarian cortex seen at early second-look laparoscopy six weeks later. No adhesions are encountered the majority of the time when using permanent suture following microlaser ovarian wedge resection if adequate hemostasis is obtained.

Excising an ovarian cyst without the microscope

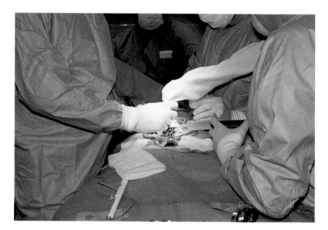

Figure 4.67 The hand piece may be used with optic loupes with the articulating arm covered by a plastic video drape or a sterile orthopedic stocking.

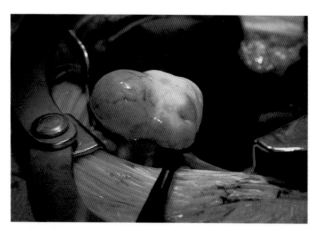

Figure 4.68 A small benign ovarian cyst is brought into the surgical field.

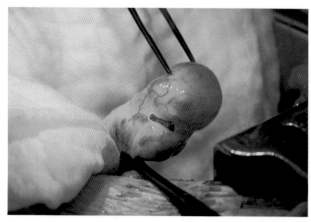

Figure 4.69 Moistened non-woven laparotomy sponges are used to insulate vital intra-abdominal structures.

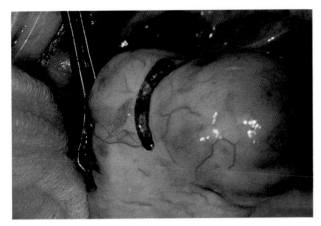

Figure 4.70 Using 35 watts superpulse with a hand piece, high power densities are obtained which allows the cyst to be excised rapidly.

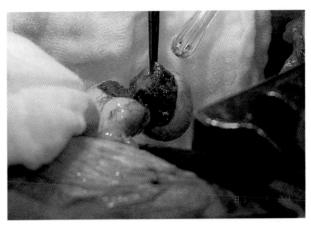

Figure 4.71 Smoke evacuation is done with the suction tip and a smoke evacuator.

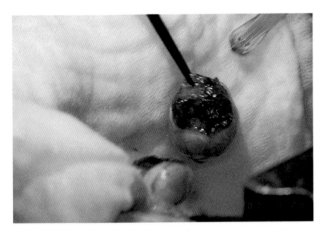

Figure 4.72 The cyst is removed in its entirety with hemostasis obtained with cautery.

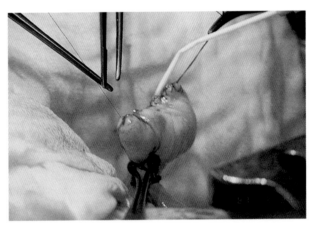

Figure 4.73 Using the microsurgical technique with optic loupes for magnification the ovary is closed with 4-0 Surgilon times two and 6-0 Surgilon.

Microlaser excision of pelvic adhesions

Figure 4.74 The pelvic adhesions overlying the left ovary are grasped with the carbide-tipped pick-ups. Note the laparotomy sponges in the background with the He–Ne aiming beam in the foreground. Continuous 35 watts superpulse is used with a quartz rod placed behind the adhesion to absorb the laser energy as the adhesion is excised.

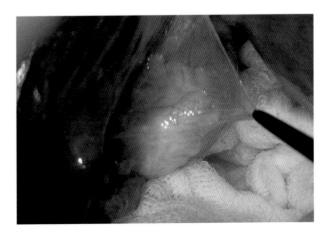

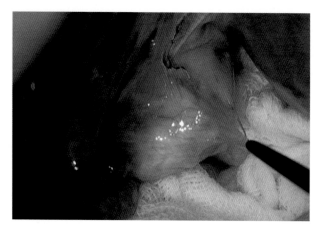

Figure 4.75 The adhesion is excised by directing the CO_2 laser's energy over the quartz rod.

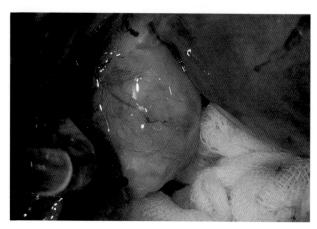

Figure 4.76 The beam may be defocused at 10 watts; using circumferential motions, the remaining surface adhesions on the ovary may be removed.

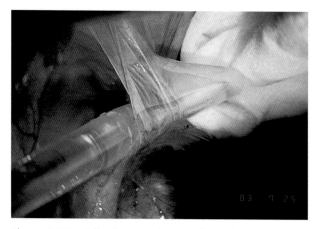

Figure 4.77 Adhesions are best excised whenever possible at the origin and insertion, again using 35 watts superpulse and a 0.2 mm spot.

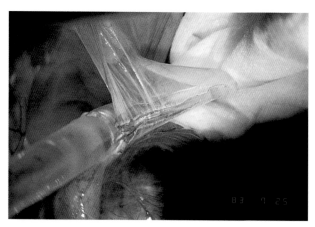

Figure 4.78 The quartz rod acts as a backstop as the laser is activated and the base of the adhesion is vaporized.

Microlaser indirect vaporization of pelvic adhesions

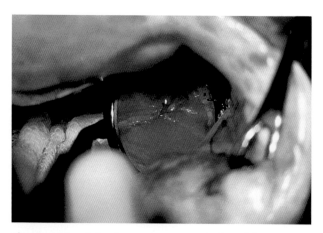

Figure 4.79 Adhesions are commonly found between the ovary and the lateral pelvic wall. The molybdenum mirror is used to visualize the adhesions, and the laser is set at 10 watts with a defocused beam.

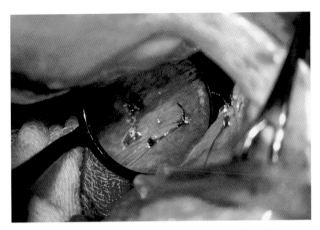

Figure 4.80 Using circumferential motion the adhesions are vaporized with traction used on the ovarian ligament to facilitate completion of the procedure.

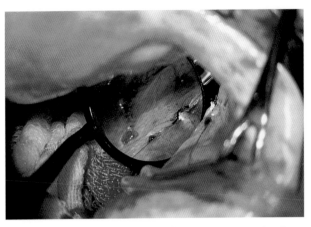

Figure 4.81 The majority of adhesions are vaporized with further lasering.

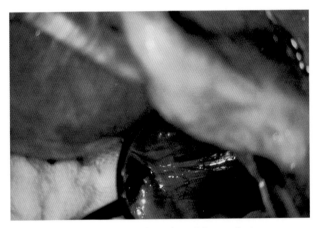

Figure 4.82 A quartz rod is placed beneath the insertion of the adhesion for this patient with the mirror used to visualize the pathology. Continuous 35 watts superpulse is used with the quartz rod to absorb the laser's energy.

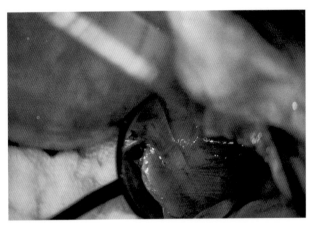

Figure 4.83 By reflecting laser energy into the mirror, the adhesion is vaporized at its insertion using the quartz rod as a backstop.

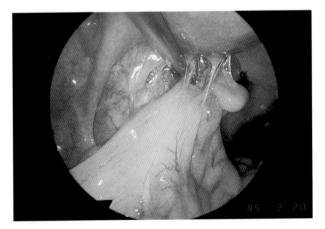

Figure 4.84 Early second-look laparoscopy six weeks post-operatively shows recurrence of filmy adhesions commonly found in the posterior cul-de-sac from the epiploic fat to the posterior uterus following previous microlaser surgery.

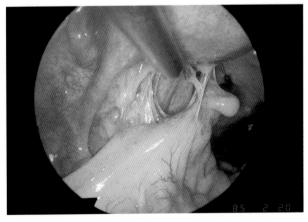

Figure 4.85 Using blunt dissection with the probe, these adhesions are easily lysed.

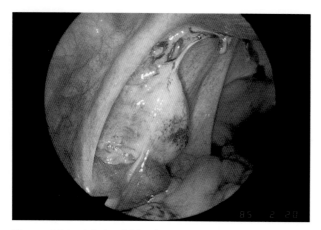

Figure 4.86 Minimal bleeding is encountered as the adnexa is mobilized.

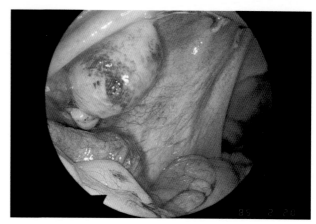

Figure 4.87 The adnexa is completely free after mobilization following early second-look laparoscopy with lysis of the filmy adhesions following microlaser laparotomy.

Microlaser fimbrioplasty

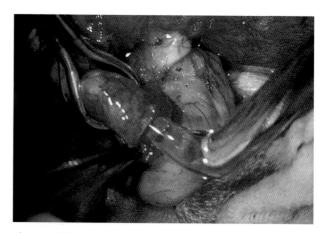

Figure 4.88 A narrow serosal collar is seen constricting the fimbria for this patient. A quartz rod is inserted into the partially patent tube with a Babcock clamp used to grasp the tube.

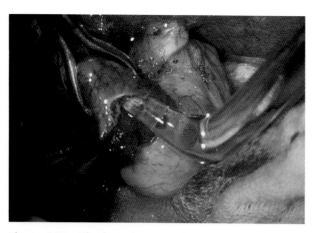

Figure 4.89 The laser is set at 35 watts superpulse, with a 0.2 mm spot, and a laser incision is made over the quartz rod.

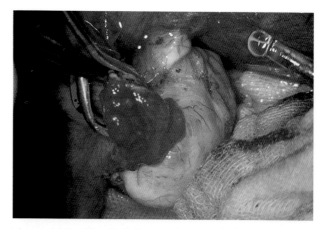

Figure 4.90 The fimbriae are freed with the serosa sutured back upon itself with 6-0 Surgilon or 8-0 Nylon.

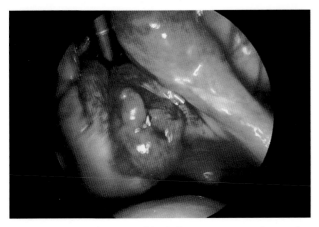

Figure 4.91 Early second-look laparoscopy at six weeks shows the tube to be patent with healthy-appearing fimbria and no further adhesion reformation.

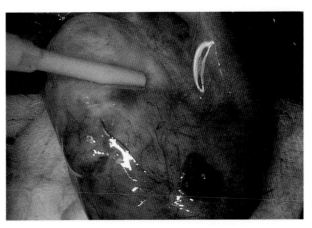

Figure 4.92 This patient had a small dimple for tubal patency with approximately 25% of the fimbriae visualized. Adhesions connected the tube to the ovary and constricted the tubal orifice.

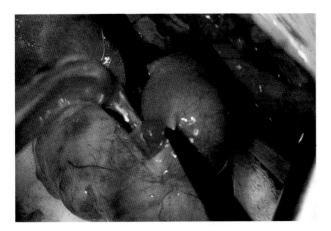

Figure 4.93 A quartz rod is inserted and the serosal portion of the tube grasped with carbide-tipped forceps.

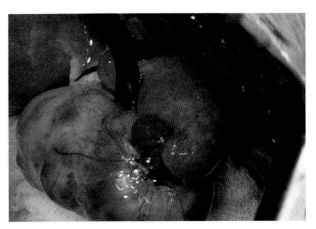

Figure 4.94 Using 35 watts superpulse with a focused beam, the incision is made over the quartz rod to open the tube.

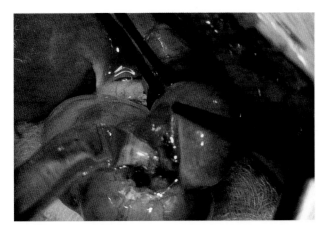

Figure 4.95 The dissection continues using the quartz rod and the laser until the tubal mucosa is everted.

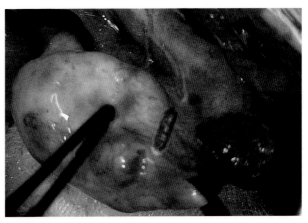

Figure 4.96 The adhesions between the ovary and tube are vaporized directly using the 35 watt power setting.

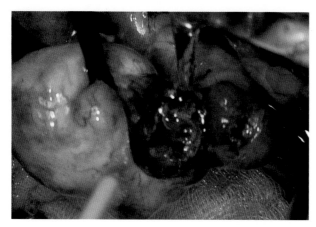

Figure 4.97 The tube is freed with more fimbriae visualized.

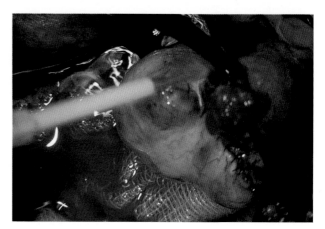

Figure 4.98 The ovarian defect is closed with 4-0 Surgilon taking care to return the anatomy to its normal place.

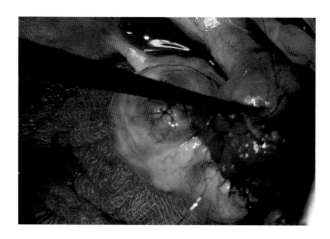

Figure 4.99 The serosa suture is back upon itself again with 6-0 Surgilon, thus a cuff fimbrioplasty is completed.

Microlaser neosalpingostomy

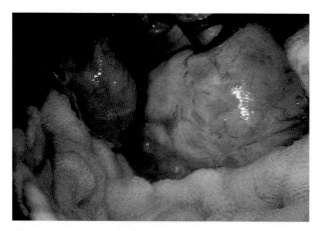

Figure 4.100 Distal tubal occlusion is noted; the dimple is seen with the He–Ne beam adjacent to it.

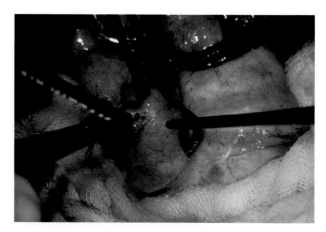

Figure 4.101 35 Watts superpulse is used to make a stellate incision into the tube.

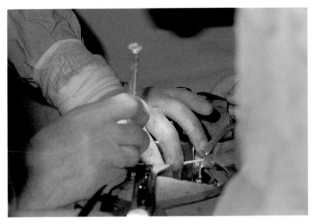

Figure 4.102 A 90° quartz rod is brought into the field.

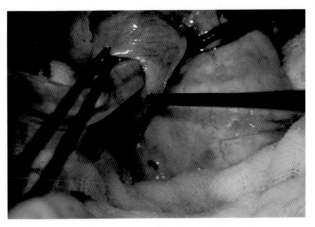

Figure 4.103 The quartz rod is inserted into the opening to further facilitate continuation of the stellate incision.

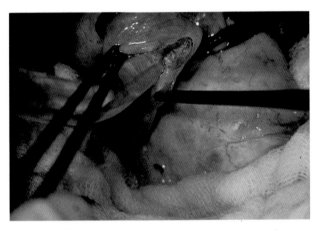

Figure 4.104 Note that the He–Ne beam is aimed at the tip of the quartz rod with traction and counter-traction used to separate the tissue.

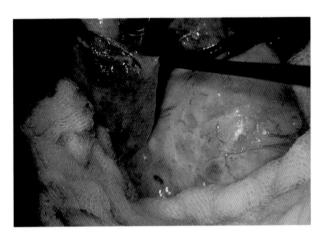

Figure 4.105 The laser has been used to extend the incision.

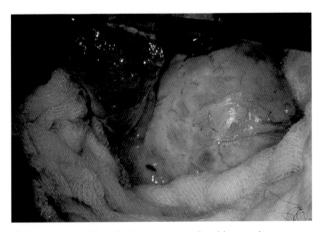

Figure 4.106 The fimbriae appear healthy as the serosa is everted.

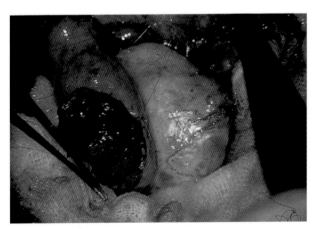

Figure 4.107 The serosa is sutured with the microsurgical technique using 8-0 Nylon.

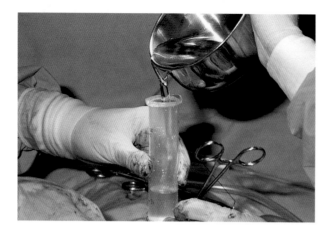

Figure 4.108 Prior to the introduction of Interceed, Gore-Tex® and Seprafilm, Hyskon was commonly used to help prevent tubal adhesions.

Laser myomectomy

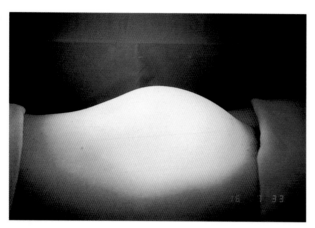

Figure 4.109 A large uterine fibroid is seen externally on this patient who had been advised to have a hysterectomy for five years and refused. She had hydronephrosis, but wished to maintain her reproductive potential.

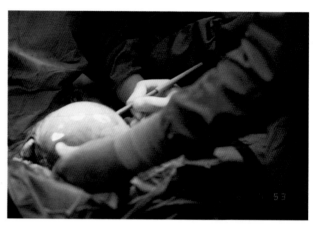

Figure 4.110 A vertical incision is made with a scalpel exposing the uterine myoma. The fibroid is palpated, outlined, and marked with a sterile marking pen.

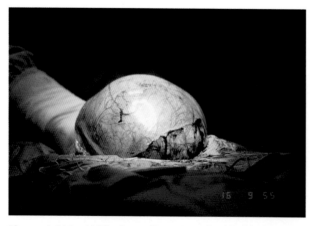

Figure 4.111 With sharp dissection, the bladder flap is taken down.

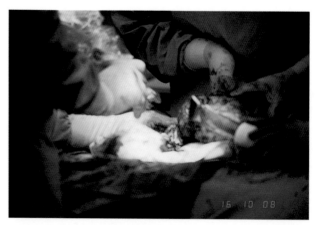

Figure 4.112 The hand piece is then used with 35 watts superpulse and the smoke evacuator near the laser impact site. The previously marked incision is vaporized, using traction and counter-traction, and a straight quartz rod under the lasered myoma attachments to facilitate fibroid removal.

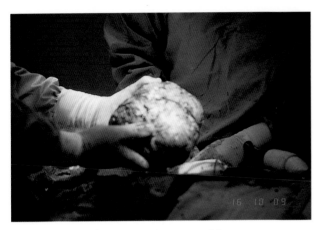

Figure 4.113 The myoma is removed intact.

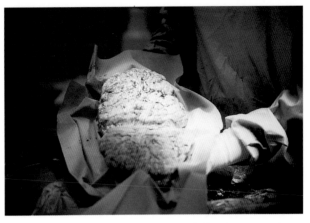

Figure 4.114 The myoma is incised showing no red degeneration.

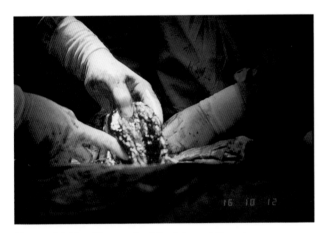

Figure 4.115 The vertical incision of the uterus anteriorly is closed with two layers of continuous 2-0 Surgilon and a serosal layer of 4-0 Surgilon.

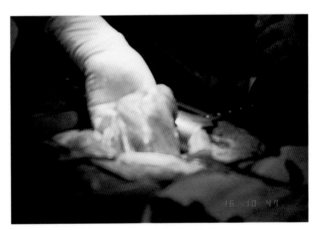

Figure 4.116 The uterus appears to be a fairly normal size after completion of the procedure.

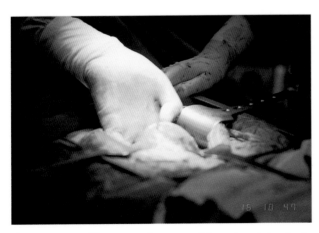

Figure 4.117 The uterus is returned into the abdominal cavity.

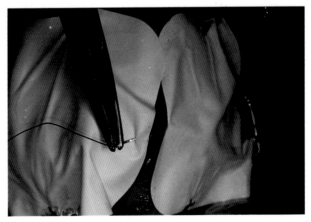

Figure 4.118 Gore-Tex® is sutured to the fundus of the uterus with a single layer of non-absorbable 2-0 Surgilon. The distal portions of the patch are sutured with absorbable 4-0 Vicryl to the uterine serosa.

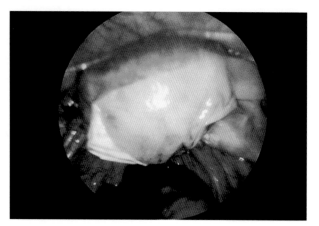

Figure 4.119 In another myomectomy patient, on early second-look laparoscopy (six weeks post-operatively), minimal adhesions are encountered on the Gore-Tex® patch.

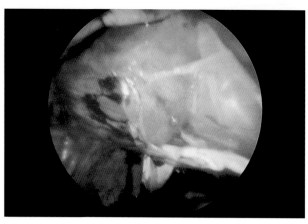

Figure 4.120 By removing the permanent Surgilon suture, the patch can be easily peeled from the uterine serosa.

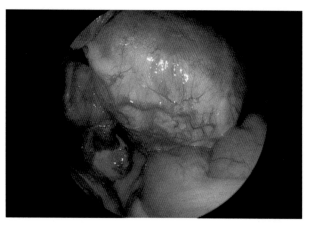

Figure 4.121 Prior to the introduction of Gore-Tex®, an omental graft was used. Often, epiploic fat adhesions to the graft were found.

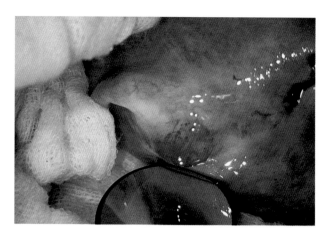

Figure 4.122 Smaller uterine fibroids may be vaporized directly or indirectly by reflecting the CO_2 laser off the molybdenum mirror to strike the pathology perpendicularly.

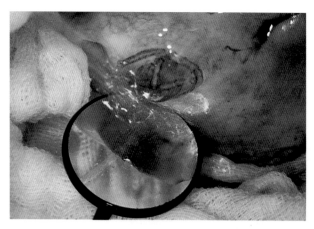

Figure 4.123 The myoma is outlined with the laser using 35 watts superpulse and a finely focused spot.

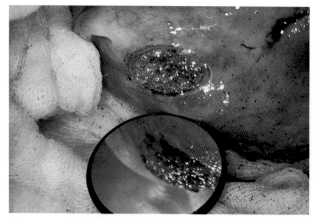

Figure 4.124 The myoma is vaporized. The defect may be covered with Gore-Tex® if shallow, or sutured first with Surgilon, if deep.

Microlaser metroplasty

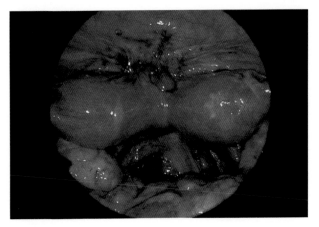

Figure 4.125 A true bicornuate uterus with endometriosis stage IV as viewed through the laparoscope.

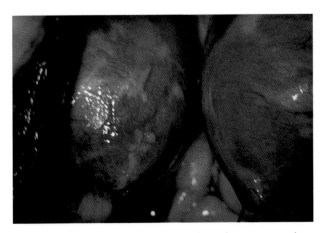

Figure 4.126 At the time of microlaser laparotomy, the uterine horns are sutured with traction sutures of 2-0 Surgilon.

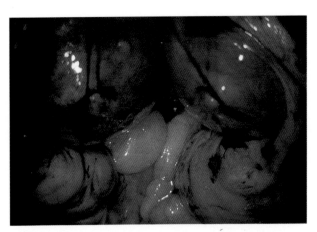

Figure 4.127 The traction sutures are noted as the endometriosis is vaporized directly and indirectly, using a defocused beam at 10 watts.

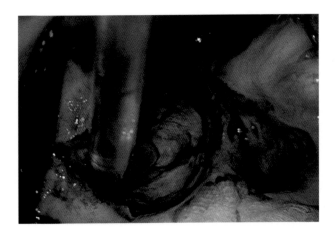

Figure 4.128 Dilute pitressin (10 units/30 cc) is injected into the medial aspect of each horn which is then marked with a sterile marking pen and the laser incision performed. The endometrial cavity is usually entered near the cervix, and a 45° angled quartz rod is placed into the uterine cavity. The laser incision is extended over the quartz rod.

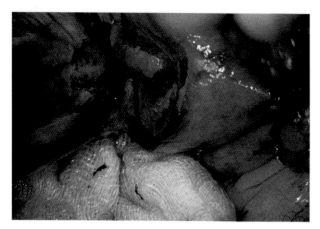

Figure 4.129 Note the hemostasis obtained with the laser; there is no bleeding on the moistened laparotomy sponge placed in the cul-de-sac.

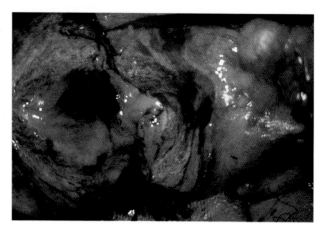

Figure 4.130 Two layers of 2-0 Surgilon are used to re-approximate the uterine cavity. Each suture is placed at the base of the two cornuae, one anteriorly, one posteriorly, and sutured deeply until the apex of the fundus is reached. In the same direction, the suture is continued and becomes superficial to be tied at the base upon completing full length from anterior to posterior and vice versa.

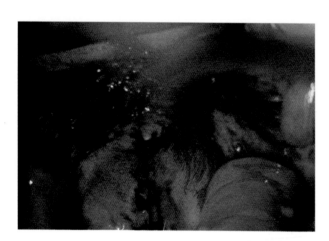

Figure 4.131 The uterine cavities are approximated and 2-0 or 4-0 Surgilon is then placed through the serosa. The round ligaments are plicated anteriorly and the ovarian ligaments plicated posteriorly.

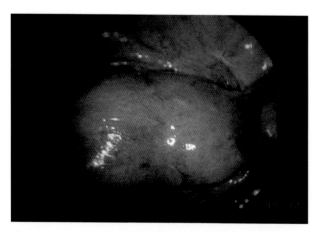

Figure 4.132 Early second-look laparoscopy shows complete uterine healing with a minimum of adhesions. Adhesions are less likely to form if excellent hemostasis is obtained at the time of metroplasty.

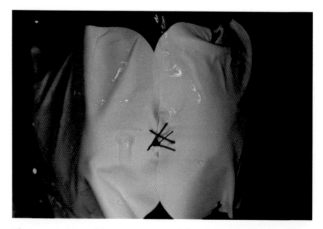

Figure 4.133 If hemostasis is difficult to obtain, a Gore-Tex® patch, placed over the uterine incision, is helpful to reduce the risk of further adhesion formation.

Microlaser removal of cornual polyps

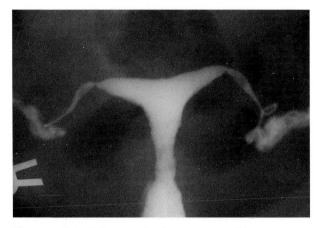

Figure 4.134 Prior to microlaser surgery, this hysterosalpingogram was obtained on a patient who was known to have fibroids and extensive endometriosis. She was deemed inoperable by her previous gynecologist. Note the large bilateral cornual polyps seen on X-ray.

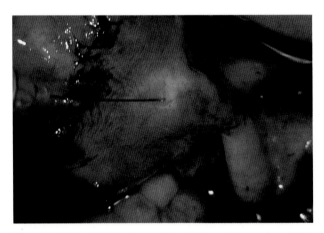

Figure 4.135 At the time of laparotomy the endometrial implants were vaporized and a myomectomy performed. Dilute pitressin (10 units/30 cc of saline) was injected over the swollen cornual polyps.

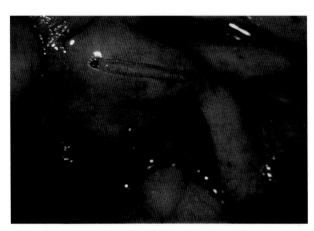

Figure 4.136 Using 35 watts superpulse with a focused beam, a linear incision was made over the swollen cornuae.

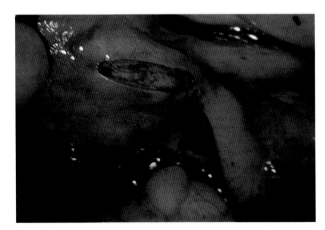

Figure 4.137 Using traction and counter-traction, the incision was extended.

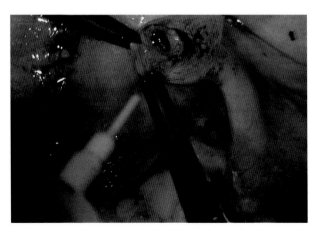

Figure 4.138 Exposure of the cornual polyp.

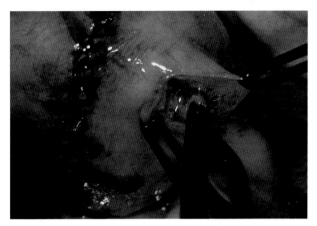

Figure 4.139 The polyp was grasped with a carbide-tipped micro-Allis clamp. The laser was used to excise the polyp at its base.

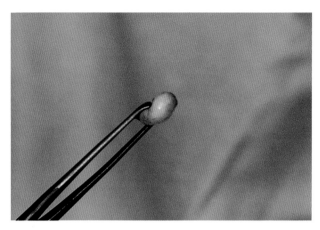

Figure 4.140 The polyps were completely excised bilaterally.

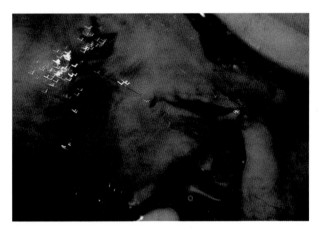

Figure 4.141 The cornuae were closed with deep 4-0 Surgilon.

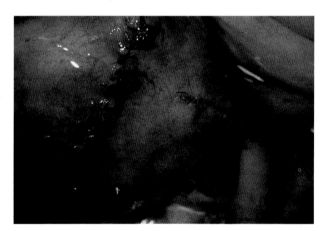

Figure 4.142 6-0 Surgilon was used to re-approximate the serosa.

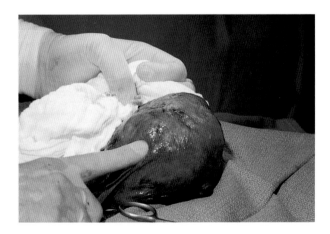

Figure 4.143 The patient was advised to avoid pregnancy for six months, and spontaneously conceived the following month. She delivered at term. Cesarean section was performed due to the extensive myomectomy. At the time of surgery no adhesion formation on the uterus or the cornual area was seen.

Microlaser tubal reanastomosis

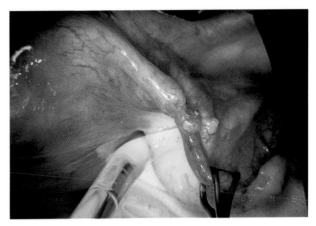

Figure 4.144 A mid-segment tubal sterilization is seen with a quartz rod placed beneath the scar tissue. The laser is used to vaporize the tissue at the tip, enabling the quartz rod to be placed directly underneath the tube.

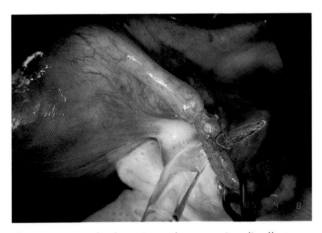

Figure 4.145 The laser is used to vaporize distally to the obstruction over the quartz rod, taking care not to extend the laser energy into the mucosa.

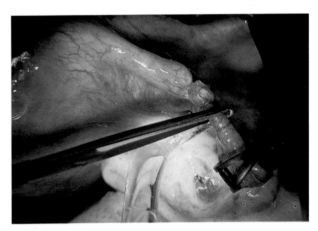

Figure 4.146 Sharp dissection is used to excise the mucosa with Iris scissors.

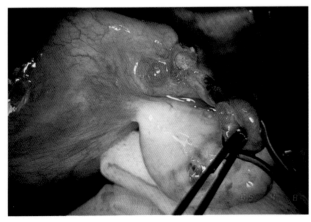

Figure 4.147 The healthy tubal mucosa is visualized. The remainder of the proximal obstruction is similarly excised with the laser.

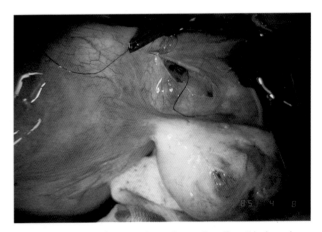

Figure 4.148 A base suture of 4-0 Surgilon is placed into the mesosalpinx. It is quite important to avoid tension at this site so that the tube may heal completely. Just beneath the tubal muscularis, a second base suture of 6-0 Surgilon is placed.

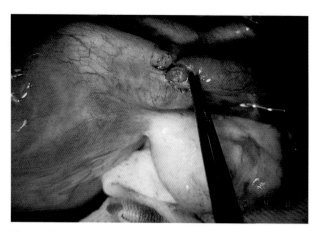

Figure 4.149 The muscularis is approximated with four sutures of 8-0 Nylon.

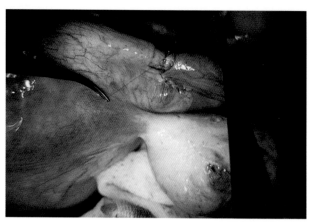

Figure 4.150 To close the serosa, an 8-0 Nylon suture is placed at the anterior base of the tubal incision and tied. The free end is left hanging.

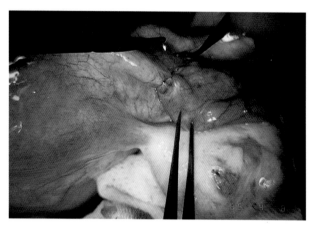

Figure 4.151 The needle is brought posteriorly through the mesosalpinx.

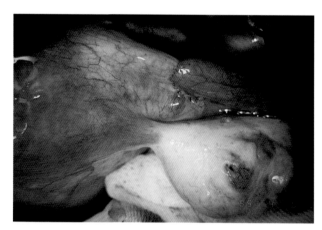

Figure 4.152 A continuous suture is started, approximating the tubal serosa, which is completed and then tied at the base.

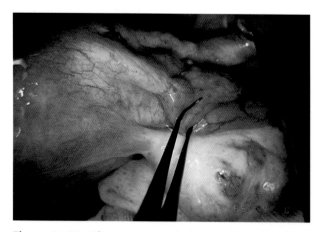

Figure 4.153 The reanastomosis is complete when the suture is finished.

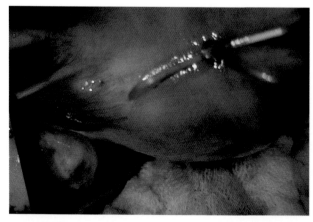

Figure 4.154 For tubal cornual reanastomosis a Buxton clamp is placed around the uterine cervix, a butterfly needle inserted into the uterine cavity, and blue dye injected. The bulge from the isthmic portion of the tube is visualized.

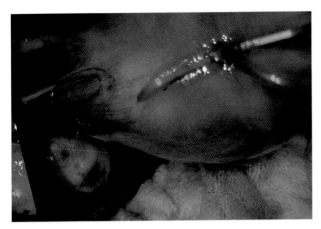

Figure 4.155 The laser is used at 35 watts superpulse, in circumferential fashion, to open the scarred area on the uterus after dilute pitressin was inserted.

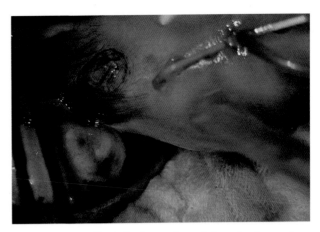

Figure 4.156 The isthmic portion of the tube is nearly entered.

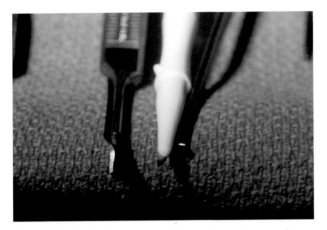

Figure 4.157 A sharp ophthalmic knife is best used to remove the remaining isthmic portion of the tube.

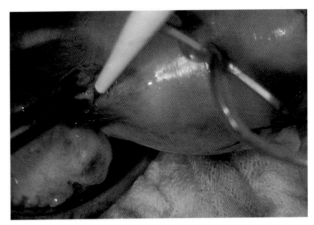

Figure 4.158 A carbide-tipped micro-Allis clamp is used to grasp the remaining portion of the tube as the eye knife is used.

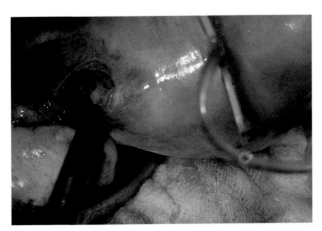

Figure 4.159 The tubal opening is seen as dye is injected.

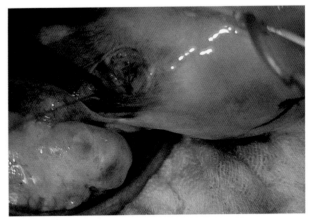

Figure 4.160 A base suture of 4-0 Surgilon is used to approximate the distal portion of the tube to the uterus.

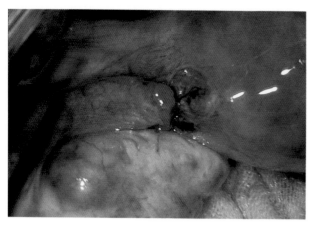

Figure 4.161 It is most important to minimize the stress on the suture and approximate the tube as closely as possible to the uterus using the 4-0 Surgilon base suture.

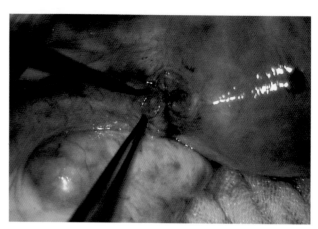

Figure 4.162 A suture of 6-0 Surgilon is placed through the tubal muscularis to the uterus.

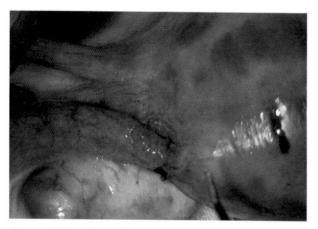

Figure 4.163 8-0 Nylon sutures are placed through the muscularis.

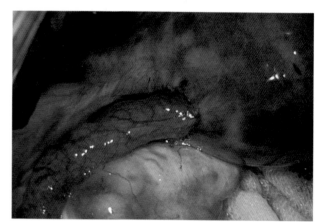

Figure 4.164 The serosal layer is closed with 6-0 Surgilon or 8-0 Nylon.

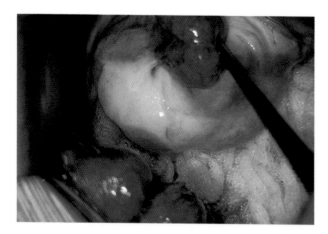

Figure 4.165 Methylene blue dye is injected to confirm tubal patency at the conclusion of the procedure.

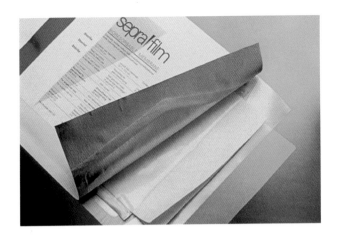

Figure 4.166 Seprafilm is useful for microlaser surgery when it is difficult to obtain hemostasis. Myomectomy and metroplasty may result in some oozing from the suture line, particularly when the pitressin wears off. It is important to dry the field and your gloves prior to placing the Seprafilm, still in its paper holder, into the field. When the membrane is located properly, the paper holder is removed, and the Seprafilm moistened. The advantage of this adhesive barrier is its absorption as opposed to Gore-Tex® (courtesy of Genzyme, Inc.).

BIBLIOGRAPHY

Badaway ZA, Elbakry M, Baggish MS: Comparative study of continuous and pulsed CO_2 laser on tissue healing and fertility outcome in tubal anastomosis. *Fertil Steril* **47**:843–9, 1987.

Baggish MS, Chong AP: Carbon dioxide laser microsurgery of the uterine tube. *Obstet Gynecol* **58**:111–22, 1981.

Baggish MS, Chong AP: Intra-abdominal surgery with the CO_2 laser. *J Reprod Med* **28**:269–76, 1983.

Bailey H, Ott M, Hartendorp P: Aggressive surgical management for advanced colorectal endometriosis. *Dis Colon Rectum* **37**:747–53, 1994.

Barbot J, Parent B, Dubuisson J, et al: A clinical study of the CO_2 laser and electrosurgery for adhesiolysis in 172 cases followed by early second-look laparoscopy. *Fertil Steril* **48**:140–9, 1987.

Bellina JH: Gynecology and the laser. *Contemp Obstet Gynecol* **4**:24–31, 1974.

Bellina J: Microsurgery of the fallopian tube with the carbon dioxide laser: analysis of 230 cases with two year follow-up. *Lasers Surg Med* **3**:255–67, 1983.

Bruhat MA, Mage G: Pregnancy following salpingostomy: comparison between CO_2 laser and electrosurgery procedures. *Fertil Steril* **40**:472–77, 1983.

Chong AP, Baggish MS: Management of pelvic endometriosis by means of intra-abdominal carbon dioxide laser. *Fertil Steril* **41**:14–23, 1984.

Cropp CS, Cowell PLD, Rock JA: Failure of tube closure following laser salpingostomy for ampullary tubal ectopic pregnancy. *Fertil Steril* **48**:887–9, 1987.

Daniell J, Diamond M, McLaughlin D, et al: Clinical results of terminal salpingostomy with the use of the CO_2 laser: report of the intra-abdominal laser study group. *Fertil Steril* **45**:175–8, 1986.

Diamond MP, Daniell JF, Martin DC, et al: Pelvic adhesions at early second-look laparoscopy following carbon dioxide laser surgical procedures. *Fertil Steril* **42**:39–43, 1984.

Diamond D, Daniell J, Martin D, Feste J, Vaughn W, McLaughlin D: Tubal patency and pelvic adhesions at early second-look laparoscopy following intra-abdominal use of the carbon dioxide laser: initial report of the intra-abdominal laser study group. *Fertil Steril* **42**:717–23, 1984.

Diamond M, Seprafilm Adhesion Study Group: Reduction of adhesions after uterine myomectomy by Seprafilm membrane (HAL-F): a blinded, prospective, randomized, multicenter clinical study. *Fertil Steril* **66**:904–10, 1996.

Diamond M, Sepracoat Adhesion Study Group: Reduction of de novo postsurgical adhesions by intraoperative precoating with Sepracoat (HAL-C) solution: a prospective, randomized, blinded, placebo-controlled, multicenter study. The Sepracoat Adhesion Study Group. *Fertil Steril* **69**: 1067–74, 1998.

Fayez JA, McComb JS, Harper MA: Comparison of tubal microsurgery with the CO_2 laser and the unipolar micro-electrode. *Fertil Steril* **40**:476–82, 1983.

Feste JR: Laser therapy for endometriosis, adhesions, and tubal disease. In McLaughlin DS (ed.): *Lasers in Gynecology.* Philadelphia, J.B. Lippincott, pp 149–68, 1991.

Filmar S, Gomel V, McComb PF: The effectiveness of CO_2 laser and electromicrosurgery in adhesiolysis: a comparative study. *Fertil Steril* **45**:407–11, 1986.

McLaughlin DS: Microlaser myomectomy technique to enhance reproductive potential: a preliminary report. *Lasers Surg Med* **2**:107–13, 1982.

McLaughlin DS: Laser instrumentation for intra-abdominal microlaser gynecological surgery. *J Clin Laser Med Surg* **2**:193–201, 1982.

McLaughlin DS: Advanced surgical instrumentation needed for intra-abdominal application of the carbon dioxide laser in reproductive biology. *Lasers Surg Med* **2**:241–52, 1983.

McLaughlin DS: Evaluation of adhesion reformation by early second-look laparoscopy following microlaser ovarian wedge resection. *Fertil Steril* **42**:531–7, 1984.

McLaughlin DS: Successful pregnancy outcome following removal of bilateral cornual polyps by microsurgical linear salpingostomy with the aid of the CO_2 laser. *Fertil Steril* **42**:938–41, 1984.

McLaughlin DS: Metroplasty and myomectomy with the CO_2 laser for maximizing the preservation of normal tissue and minimizing blood loss. *J Reprod Med* **30**:1–7, 1985.

McLaughlin DS: Current uses of the laser for fertility—promoting procedures. *Lasers Surg Med* **5**:539–61, 1985.

McLaughlin DS: Instruments necessaires pour une microlaser de surete. *Rev Fr Gynecol Obstet* **81**:47–56, 1986.

McLaughlin DS, Bonaventura LM, Jarrett JC II: Tubal reanastomosis: a comparison between microsurgical and microlaser techniques. *Microsurgery* **8**:78–87, 1987.

McLaughlin DS, Diamond MP, Daniell JF, et al: Laparoscopic assessment of ovarian healing following CO_2 laser micro-surgery: Vicryl vs Surgilon. *Microsurgery* **8**:99–112, 1987.

McLaughlin DS: Uterine and ovarian laser surgery. In: McLaughlin DS (ed.): *Lasers in Gynecology*. Philadelphia, J.B. Lippincott, pp 169–98, 1991.

Pittaway DE, Maxson WS, Daniell JF: A comparison of the CO_2 laser and electrocautery on postoperative intra-peritoneal adhesion formation in rabbits. *Fertil Steril* **40**:366–71, 1983.

Tjaden B, Schlaff W, Kimball A, Rock J: The efficacy of presacral neurectomy for the relief of midline dysmenorrhea. *Obstet Gynecol* **76**:89–91, 1990.

Tulandi T, Farag R, McInnes R, et al: Reconstructive surgery of hydrosalpinx with and without the carbon dioxide laser. *Fertil Steril* **42**:839–45, 1984.

Tulandi T, Viols G: A comparison between laser surgery and electrosurgery for bilateral hydrosalpinx: a two year follow-up. *Fertil Steril* **44**:841–52, 1985.

Tulandi T: Salpingo-ovariolysis: a comparison between laser surgery and electrosurgery. *Fertil Steril* **45**:489–97, 1986.

Tulandi T: Adhesion reformation after reproductive surgery with and without the carbon dioxide laser. *Fertil Steril* **47**:704, 1987.

Voros JI, Bellina JH, Moorehead ME, et al: Management of ectopic pregnancy by carbon dioxide laser. *J LA State Med Soc* **135**:9–12, 1984.

5 Assisted reproductive technology

Aristotle was quoted as saying, 'For any living thing that has reached its normal development and which is unmutilated, and whose mode of generation is not spontaneous, the most natural act is the production of another like itself... That is the goal toward which all things strive.'

Aristotle, quoted in: On the Relationship of Parents and Children. *Ethics Reprod Tech* **132**:133–4, 1992.

Assisted reproductive technology (ART) attempts to achieve this goal using currently evolving technology.

Indications for IVF and GIFT

Patients under age 35, who have failed conventional therapy, and those who may have diminishing ovarian reserve should be considered candidates for assisted reproductive technology (ART). Depending on the individual program's success rate, IVF may still be preferred to GIFT even when accessible and patent tubes are available, especially if male factor is involved. However, a logical protocol to consider would be to recommend:

- IVF for the treatment of:
  - Inaccessible, absent, or blocked fallopian tubes
  - Need to document fertilization for less than optimal gametes, especially for diminished ovarian reserve
  - Need for a micromanipulation procedure (intra-cytoplasmic sperm injection—ICSI or assisted hatching)
  - Requires at least one functioning ovary, uterus, and spermatozoa (husband or donor).
- GIFT for the treatment of:
  - Endometriosis
  - Ovulation disorders
  - Immunologic disease states (sperm antibodies)
  - Idiopathic
  - Requires at least one functioning, accessible ovary and fallopian tube, and normal spermatozoa (husband or donor).

Prior to considering an ART cycle, it may be wise to prescreen the infertile couple in various ways.

Assess the patient's ovarian reserve

Reproductive potential declines with age and may be seen as longer duration to conceive with a lessened chance to produce a livebirth. The uniformly successful oocyte donation pregnancy rates, at any recipient's age, indicate that the non-ovarian components of the reproductive system are not severely affected by age. The decline in reproductive potential due to diminished oocyte quality and further follicular depletion is termed diminished ovarian reserve.

A Day 3 follicle-stimulating hormone (FSH) level greater than 25 mIU/ml (Binax assay) indicates a very poor prognosis for conception and donor egg should be considered. Scott analyzed 758 IVF cycles and found that the greatest chance of success was in women whose basal FSH was less than 15 mIU/ml. A Day 3 FSH level greater than 15 mIU/ml combined with an estradiol level greater than 75 pg/ml often predicts a lower response, which may indicate the need to use a low responder protocol combined with assisted hatching to increase the chance for conception and subsequent implantation.

To help further assess subtle changes in ovarian reserve, the clomiphene citrate challenge test (CCT) may be helpful. With this test a basal FSH is drawn on Day 3, then daily clomiphene 100 mg is administered Day 5 through 9, and another FSH is drawn on Day 10. An abnormal test is determined by an elevated FSH on Day 10. Scott found the incidence of an abnormal CCT to be: 3% under age 30, 7% for ages 30–34, 10% for those 35–39, and 26% for those women over 40 years of age. In his study, pregnancy rates were 9% for those women with a diminished ovarian reserve versus 43% for those with a normal ovarian function. CCT appears to be two to three times more sensitive than basal FSH to detect declining ovarian reserve. Only seven of 23 patients who had an elevated Day 10 FSH in Scott's CCT study had an elevated Day 3 FSH.

Since female smoking increases the risk of miscarriage and halves the chance for conception, all women undergoing an ART treatment cycle should be advised to stop smoking. Those who persist generally require about a third more ampoules (amps) of FSH to obtain an adequate response.

Semen analysis

If white blood cells are present, antibiotics and frequent ejaculation should help to optimize the spermatozoa at the time of retrieval. If the sperm morphology is less than 4% by strict criteria, ICSI may be considered. Sperm morphology may be enhanced by recommending the male to stop smoking and ingest 1 gram Vitamin C daily.

Antisperm antibodies

If present in follicular fluid, additional oocyte washes with the supplementation of increased numbers of sperm may be helpful. If male antibodies are present, additional sperm may be added after the specimen is recovered from ejaculation into antibody-free serum in culture medium. In severe cases, ICSI may be advised.

Chlamydia antibodies

A reduction in pregnancy rates and increase in miscarriages have been attributed to chronic endometrial infection or scarring from prior infection. Zithromax is currently the antibiotic of choice for both partners.

Trial embryo transfer

The pregnancy rate is positively affected by a trial transfer prior to the ovulation induction; it also facilitates the actual embryo transfer. Pregnancy rates drop from 20% to 3% for those patients who had a retained embryo in the catheter following a difficult transfer.

Check for uterine and/or tubal abnormalities

Precycle ultrasound at the time of trial transfer should help to detect endometrial polyps or a submucous myoma which could negatively affect embryo implantation. The sensitivity of ultrasound

may be enhanced by injecting saline (saline infusion sonohysterogram—SIS). Some authors have recommended routine hysteroscopy prior to the ART cycle. They suggest that a septate uterus should be treated prior to ART in order to reduce the chance of miscarriage. Maternal exposure to diethylstilbestrol in utero reduces the chance of pregnancy by half, particularly with a T-shaped cavity, but reverts to normal when the cavity was small, but shaped normally.

Hydrosalpinges are associated with a reduced chance of implantation and an increased chance of pregnancy loss. These should be treated by salpingostomy or salpingectomy prior to a treatment cycle. By ultrasound evaluation of in vitro fertilization with embryo transfer (IVF-ET) patients the frequency of hydrosalpinges appears to be 10–13%. However, the incidence rises to 25–30% when the diagnosis is based on hysterosalpingogram (HSG), laparoscopy, or laparotomy. Atri reported that only 34% of patients with hydrosalpinges were identified by ultrasound prior to HSG. Recent studies demonstrated a reduction in pregnancy rate per retrieval for those with tubal disease who had a hydrosalpinx (10% vs 23%). The mechanism of action appears to be the negative effect on endometrial integrin expression by the fluid in the hydrosalpinges. After treatment, the pregnancy rate increased to 38%.

Treat endometriosis

Eradicating endometriosis prior to an ART cycle appears to enhance the chance of fertilization and implantation by removing the inhibiting effects of the disease. This seems to be particularly true if a gonadotropin agonist is used after surgery, prior to controlled ovarian hyperstimulation. The mechanism of action is postulated to be mediated through uterine integrins, which are cell adhesion molecules which have alpha and beta extracellular receptors. Usually, there is a three day window of implantation, as 2/3 integrins overlap to facilitate implantation. If the endometrium fails to produce the appropriate integrin, at the right time, an occult defect in uterine receptivity occurs, and the chance for implantation is diminished. Further research is ongoing to facilitate the chance of embryonic implantation following ART (Table 5.1).

Stimulation protocols

The use of gonadotropin agonists with FSH therapy has doubled the pregnancy rate, reduced the cancellation rate due to premature luteinizing hormone (LH) surge, and improved scheduling for oocyte retrieval.

Table 5.1 **Clinical ART pregnancy statistics while the author was a partner at the Indianapolis Fertility Center (1986–95)**

GIFT	44.4%	948/2135
IVF	20.8%	254/1222
ZIFT	38.7%	143/370

Effect of Lupron down regulation (after 4/89)

	Pre-day 21 Lupron		Post-day 21 Lupron	
GIFT	35%	210/596	48%	740/1544
IVF	14%	57/396	24%	198/827
ZIFT	50%	1/2	39%	142/368

Clinical outcome since Lupron (4/89–1/94)

Ectopics	5%	45/927
Miscarriages	20%	183/927
Stillborns	1%	11/927
Deliveries	74%	688/927
Singletons	49%	455/927
Twins	18%	165/927
Triplets	6%	58/927
Quads	1%	9/927
Quints	0.1%	1/927

- The protocols for normal responders are:
  - Day 21 Lupron 1 mg decreasing to 0.5 mg with the start of FSH therapy 225 units per day on 'Day 3'
  - Day 21 Lupron 0.5 mg decreasing to 0.25 mg with the start of FSH therapy 300 units per day on 'Day 3'
- Protocols for high responders (polycystic ovaries or patients who have previously experienced ovarian hyperstimulation syndrome (OHSS))
  - A low-dose oral contraceptive is started the previous cycle, for 25 days
  - Lupron 0.1 cc is started Day 21, with FSH 150 units per day
  - If the estradiol rapidly rises with multiple small follicles, the patient may coast up to 2 days with no deleterious effects.
- For known or anticipated low responders, the microdose Lupron flare is used in conjunction with IVF and assisted hatching:
  - Oral contraceptives are prescribed for 9–21 days
  - 3 days later Lupron 40 micrograms b.i.d. is started with FSH 3 amps b.i.d. until human chorionic gonadotropin (hCG) is given
  - The embryos are hatched; tetracycline 250 mg q.i.d. and methylprednisolone 16 mg q.d. are administered for four days, starting the day of retrieval.

Patients are warned that the chance of cancellation due to a poor response may occur up to 15% of the time, and donor egg advised.

Diminished ovarian reserve may result from previous ovarian surgery, severe endometriosis, advancing age, or may be idiopathic. The peak estradiol and number of oocytes retrieved decline by nearly half at age 40 as compared to women aged 30.

The strategies to improve the ovarian response for poor responders include: decreasing the Lupron dose, increasing the FSH dose, using the Lupron flare protocol, or combining clomiphene with FSH. Adding more than 4 amps of FSH usually does not appear helpful, however decreasing the amount of Lupron with the microdose regimen stimulates endogenous FSH to aid in the recruitment of oocytes and subsequent estradiol production. Pretreatment with oral contraceptives enhances the response in poor responders with a normal FSH level, eliminates the previous corpus luteum, and prevents subsequent premature LH surge with ovulation induction. Schoolcraft was able to achieve an average peak estradiol of 1295 pg/ml with 11 oocytes retrieved and an ongoing pregnancy rate of 50% for his group of low responders.

The timing of hCG administration appears to be more flexible for those being treated with the long protocol (Day 21 Lupron) but more critical for the short protocol (Lupron flare).

Luteal phase support appears to be essential for those patients who have been pretreated with gonadotropin-releasing hormone analogs. Intramuscular or vaginal progesterone appears to be as effective as 2000 IU of hCG given on days 4, 8, and 12 of the luteal phase. The currently recommended progesterone therapy for luteal phase support is 50 mg i.m. daily starting the day after retrieval for 14 days. If pregnancy ensues, the dose is adjusted up 25 mg if the progesterone level is less than 20 ng/ml and down 25 mg if the progesterone level is greater than 70. Crinone progesterone gel, applied vaginally, appears to have a positive effect on implantation, and may be used instead of i.m. progesterone. Luteal phase support is generally continued until about 10 weeks' gestation.

There are several considerations to make when deciding to recommend GIFT. These include whether the laparoscopic treatment modality improves the probability of success over simpler therapies (ovulation induction and intra-uterine insemination) and whether it is superior to ultrasonic IVF-ET. The chance of delivering a child after one cycle of GIFT is significantly greater than the chance of spontaneous conception, particularly for patients with idiopathic infertility. A randomized trial demonstrated that GIFT was significantly superior to spontaneous cycle with intra-uterine insemination, and superovulation/insemination. Only a very few small prospective randomized comparative trials have been published comparing the success of GIFT with IVF-ET. If male factors are excluded, these studies have shown a higher pregnancy rate with transtubal transfer of gametes as opposed to transcervical transfer of embryos. It is apparent that quantity and quality of oocytes transferred via GIFT are important. A potential drawback of GIFT is the lessened ability to control higher-order multiple gestation. Definitely, if there is question of fertilizability of the gametes, IVF is preferred to document this potential.

Techniques

IVF

For retrieval, monitored intravenous sedation is generally used with an automated blood pressure cuff and pulse oximeter. Local anesthesia is not used due to potential embryo toxicity. Tetracycline is started for those undergoing assisted hatching. Culture media serves as the preparative solution, not betadine, which may significantly reduce the pregnancy rate. The follicles are visualized by transvaginal ultrasound, aspirated, and flushed with tissue culture media. Generally the intrafollicular pressure is limited to 100 mmHg, until the final flush when the maximum pressure (400 mmHg) is used. A double lumen needle is preferred by the author, as the follicle may be distended with the flush, which may help to dislodge the oocyte. It is vital to keep the oocytes warm after aspiration, prior to transfer to the embryology laboratory. This can be accomplished by using a heating block with 1–2 cc of tissue culture fluid in each test tube used for follicular aspiration (Figs 5.1–5.25).

For transfer, no sedation is used. The vagina is prepared and a Wallace catheter is used to aspirate the cervical mucous prior to transfer (Figs 5.26–5.30). Poindexter published that 9% of patients had embryos in the cervix or speculum after an uncomplicated transfer, which can be reduced by proper technique.

McNamee recently described a new embryo transfer technique using vigorous cervical lavage prior to embryo transfer with a Wallace catheter. He based his premise on Egbase's work in London who demonstrated a lowered pregnancy rate for those

women whose cervical mucous and catheter tips cultured positive at the time of embryo transfer. The cervical mucous is vigorously lavaged with tissue culture media, using a syringe and cannula. When the mucous is removed and no bleeding is present, a dummy trial Wallace embryo catheter is placed under abdominal ultrasound monitoring. The actual Wallace transfer catheter is then loaded and, very carefully, the embryos are placed into the uterus 1 cm prior to the uterine fundus (avoiding contact). The procedure is considered complete when the Wallace catheter is confirmed as empty by the embryologist in the laboratory.

Although bed rest is often advised by many ART programs, there has been no objective proof this is a valid recommendation. The Birmingham program, in the United Kingdom, has the patient resume normal activities immediately and has reported a 40% clinical pregnancy rate (22% implantation rate/embryo transferred).

GIFT

For laparoscopic aspiration, the peritoneal cavity is distended with carbon dioxide. Only follicular aspiration and transtubal gamete transfer are performed (Figs 5.31–5.39). For transfer, a Cook catheter is used, with a 45° angle placed at 3 cm. An air bubble separates the oocytes (up to four in total for the procedure, depending on egg quality and patient age) with 100,000 processed sperm used for each oocyte (Figs 5.40–5.43). Yee found that the success of his program was dependent on the depth of placement (>4 cm from the fimbria) and the number of oocytes replaced (4=43%, 3=23%, 2=19%, 1=0%). There was no difference in success whether one or two tubes were used, providing both were equally healthy.

Tubal ovum transfer (TOT)

Prior to the advent of GIFT, with the aid of Gary Hodgen based on his animal studies, the author initiated a program to clinically apply assisted IVF in humans. This technique was pioneered at a Catholic hospital, under the auspices of the hospital's medical–moral committee following Catholic doctrine as directed by the Pope John Center in Boston, Massachusetts. TOT is similar to GIFT, except the sperm is collected in a perforated silastic condom through natural intercourse. The birth of the first infant conceived by this technique was published in *The Lancet* in 1987. This ART procedure is unique as it was designed prospectively with ethical considerations used to mandate procedural protocols.

Results

Evolution of ART success rates		
	IVF	GIFT
Society of Assisted Reproductive Technology (Number of cases: Deliveries/Retrieval)		
1988	13,647 (12%)	3080 (21%)
1989	15,392 (14%)	3652 (23%)
1990	16,405 (14%)	3750 (22%)
1991	21,083 (15%)	4474 (27%)
1992	24,996 (17%)	4837 (27%)
1993	33,543 (18%)	4992 (28%)
1994	33,700 (21%)	4214 (29%)
1995	35,269 (23%)	3318 (27%)
1996	45,462 (26%)	2892 (29%)
Author (Number of cases: Pregnancies/Retrieval)		
1986–95	44/189 (24%)	105/243 (43%)
1998	12/28 (43%)	7/11 (64%)

Micromanipulation

Assisted hatching

IVF is often inefficient due to implantation failure. This may include abnormal embryos, suboptimal culture conditions (fewer than 25% human blastocyst will hatch in vitro), impaired uterine receptors, and abnormal zona pellucida. Assisted hatching, introduced by Cohen in 1990, was devised to facilitate embryo escape from the zona during blastocyst expansion (Figs 5.44–5.50). Although the technique still remains controversial, it is indicated for advanced maternal age, decreased ovarian reserve, increased zona thickness, previous unexplained IVF implantation failure, reduced embryo cleavage or increased fragmentation, and for in vitro oocyte maturation. The technique involves producing a 30 micrometer defect in the zona on Day 3 using acidified Tyrode's or the diode laser. The embryo transfer should be performed using a Wallace catheter with ultrasound guidance. As previously mentioned, antibiotics and cortisone are used. Cohen improved the pregnancy rate from 37% to 52% with assisted hatching. Schoolcraft reported an ongoing pregnancy rate of 64% in the hatched groups vs 19% in the non-hatched patients. For his patients over 40 years old, the results were 47% vs 11%. Both concluded that assisted hatching reduces the energy required to complete the hatching process, which is increasingly more important with declining ovarian reserve and advancing age. It also appears to resolve a relative asymmetry between the pre-embryo and the endometrium, as embryos subjected to assisted hatching implant on average of one day earlier.

ICSI

Intracytoplasmic sperm injection is the mechanical insertion of one selected spermatozoa into the cytoplasm of an oocyte. Candidates for ICSI initially were men who failed fertilization with a previous IVF cycle, but now include men who have fewer than 4% normal forms, using the strict criteria for morphology during semen analysis. Although the technique was initially reported in 1988, the first human pregnancy was reported by Palermo in 1992. ICSI may also be excellent therapy for those men with poor motility and low sperm concentration as well (Figs 5.51–5.55). Clinical pregnancy rates as high as 58%, with ongoing pregnancy rates of 50%, have been reported by the ART team at Cornell.

Critics suggests that the use of ICSI may negatively affect the genetic composition of the population, based on the Darwinian fitness theory of survival of the most fit. A review of 11 surveys of 9766 infertile men with azospermia and oligozoospermia revealed 5.8% chromosomal abnormalities (as opposed to 0.38% of phenotypically normal newborns). Thus, genetic counseling for all couples considering ICSI is considered mandatory to inform them of the possible genetic risks to their offspring. This recommendation is increasingly more important as new ART procedures are developed.

Embryo cryopreservation

The 1996 SART data report a livebirth rate of 17% per transfer of frozen embryos from non-donor eggs (Figs 5.56–5.58). The average number of embryos transferred were 3.5 in 8661 cycles. This option gives the infertile couple undergoing IVF-ET an additional chance of conception without undergoing the risks and expense of controlled ovarian hyperstimulation and ultrasonic ovarian aspiration.

Complications

OHSS

First described in 1961, this complex of symptoms include ovarian enlargement, ascites, abdominal distension, and oliguria following gonadotropin therapy. The pathophysiology is not well understood, but appears due to increased vascular permeability. The severity of the disease is related to the number of ongoing fetuses conceived. It may be prevented by withholding hCG to trigger ovulation in at risk patients. It may be preferable, however, to convert the cycle to IVF (transvaginal follicular aspiration) with cryopreservation of the embryos, and no fresh embryo transfer. This protocol has helped reduce the need to hospitalize those patients who were likely to conceive and suffer severe OHSS (Fig. 5.68).

Multiple pregnancy

The SART data for 1994 states that the multiple birth rate was 36% following ART. These pregnancies were subdivided into 28% twins, 6% triplets, and 1% higher order multiples. For 1996, The Centers for Disease Control and Prevention showed the chance of triplets and higher increased by 19% in one year, and 312% since 1980. Prevention primarily has centered on limiting the number of embryos transferred for IVF and oocytes for GIFT. As the implantation rates per embryo improve, the chance of multiple births increases. Although there is no regulation regarding the maximum number of embryos transferred in the United States, major countries in Europe, Singapore, and Australia limit the numbers of embryos transferred to two or three. Templeton and Morris analyzed the data base established by the Human Fertilization and Embryology Authority in the UK. After reviewing 44,236 cycles in 25,240 women undergoing IVF-ET, they concluded that when more than four eggs were fertilized, there was no increase in birth rate for women receiving three embryos, as opposed to two, but the multiple birth rate was significantly higher (1.6:1). Unfortunately, when uniformly applied to all patients, this unnecessarily restricts the opportunity for success to those women with reduced ovarian reserve and advancing age.

Further research into the nutritive support of growing embryos has enabled embryos to be cultured for five days. Optimistically only half of the embryos will survive between Day 3 and 5 since many normally appearing embryos are genetically abnormal or lack the glycolytic activity required to implant. Blastocyst implantation rates appear to be superior to embryos grown for three days. With this advance in embryo culturing technique, limiting embryo transfer to two blastocysts should result in excellent pregnancy rates while reducing the chance of multiple births (Figs 5.59–5.67; Table 5.2).

Table 5.2 Age-related ART pregnancy success – 1996 SART data – Fresh embryos from non-donor eggs

35 years old or younger	
Number of cycles	22,811
Pregnancies per cycle	33%
Livebirths per cycle	29%
Livebirths per retrieval	32%
Livebirths per transfer	34%
Multiple rate	43%
35–39 years old	
Number of cycles	18,361
Pregnancies per cycle	27%
Livebirths per cycle	21%
Livebirths per retrieval	25%
Livebirths per transfer	27%
Multiple rate	35%
Greater than 39 years old	
Number of cycles	8,412
Pregnancies per cycle	13%
Livebirths per cycle	9%
Livebirths per retrieval	11%
Livebirths per transfer	12%
Multiple rate	21%

Table 5.3 Assisted reproductive technologies clinical pregnancies/transfer[1]. David McLaughlin, M.D., Jeffrey Boldt, Ph.D. Assisted fertility services Community Hospital North, Indianapolis, Indiana 3/98 to 12/98

Vaginal ultrasonic oocyte retrieval	
• Day 3 Embryo transfer (6/21)	28.6%
• Day 5 Blastocyst transfer (6/7)	85.7%
Subtotal: IVF pregnancy rate (12/98)	42.8%
Laparoscopic oocyte retrieval	
• Combination IVF/GIFT (2/5)	40%
• Gamete intra-fallopian transfer (2/3)	66.7%
• Tubal ovum transfer (3/3)	100%
Subtotal: GIFT pregnancy rate (7/11)	63.6%
Total: ART pregnancy rate[2] (19/39)	48.7%

[1] One patient retrieved with no embryos available for transfer.
[2] ASRM disclaimer. 'As entry criteria are highly variable for each program, a center-by-center comparison of results is not valid.'

There appears to be much more control in limiting the number of possible conceptuses with ART than with gonadotropin therapy alone for ovulation induction. The author supervised the Pergonal conception resulting in the successful delivery of the Dilley sextuplets in 1993 after a six year history of infertility. The mother is healthy and the six children, age 5, are developing normally—both physically and mentally with no pregnancy-related sequelae. Selective reduction of those who conceive higher-order multiples has been advocated although nearly half of the time the result may be the delivery of no 'take home' babies. Recently, a maternal death occurred following the selective reduction of a patient who conceived septuplets following non-ART gonadotropin therapy. The final decision regarding the management of the higher-order multifetal pregnancy rests with the parents in conjunction with the obstetrician and neonatologists who will manage the pregnancy and newborns.

ART regulation

At least 14 nations have statutory regulation of ART procedures. Twelve specify that IVF should only be offered to couples with a stable relationship. Half have placed no limit on the number of embryos to be transferred; the other half regulate the transfer of only three embryos. Some allow for an increase for those over 35 and if neonatal facilities are available. Two countries specifically exclude GIFT from regulation, since the fertilization occurs in vivo, and the ability to control the chance of multiple birth is lessened.

Pending the outcome of the multiple civil and criminal charges filed in California for inappropriate transfer of gametes/embryos to unrelated parties, the US may soon specify procedures to insure that optimal ART care will become uniformly available to its citizens. The California case involved Luanne and John Buzzanca who used IVF with donor eggs and donor sperm. Prior to the birth of the child, Jaycee, the couple separated, and John wanted no further obligations for the child. Since neither Luanne nor John were genetically related to the child, the trial judge ruled Jaycee parentless. The appeals court reversed this decision and concluded that Luanne and John were the legal parents.

In New York, Maureen and Steven Kass had unsuccessfully undergone five egg retrieval procedures and nine embryo transfers. For the tenth procedure, Maureen's sister agreed to act as a surrogate. The couple had signed a standard consent stating that if the couple no longer wished to use the pre-embryos or couldn't agree on the disposition of them, they may be disposed of by the IVF program and used for research. When Maureen's sister did not conceive, the couple divorced. Maureen sought custody of the cryopreserved embryos, which the trial court confirmed. The appeals court overturned the ruling by stating that the provision for embryo research should be enforced.

ART programs and courts have traditionally attempted to skirt new issues raised by evolving reproductive technology by applying the sperm-donor model of secrecy to all infertility treatments and by the dependence on contracts. The California courts suggested that the legislature determine public policy regarding ART techniques for everyone, as opposed to the courts determining individual cases with specific circumstances. In 1998, the New York State Task Force on Life and the Law recommended 60 changes in professional guidelines, 30 changes in state regulation of gamete banks, and 11 new state laws. From the child-centered perspective adopted by the task force, it was determined that the woman who gives birth to the child is the child's legal mother, regardless of the genetic source of the eggs, sperm, or embryos. They also recommended that both gamete providers unanimously agree on the use of frozen embryos.

After 20 years' experience in the rapidly evolving treatment of reproductive maladies, it may be time to consider national standards and regulation for this multi-billion dollar industry in the US. Similar conclusions were reached in the UK, Australia, and Ontario more than ten years ago. The United States has been slow to conform to the rest of the world regarding these issues largely due to the prevalent belief that reproductive decisions should be left to the individual couples and their physicians.

International ART perspectives

The pathways taken to produce a livebirth differ from country to country. The ratio of ART per 100,000 population is 357 in Australia, 152 in the UK, 57 in the US, and 63 in Canada. Also, the ratio of IVF to GIFT varies: 2.7:1 in Australia, 3.3:1 in the UK, 4.2:1 in the US, and 90.8:1 in Canada. In 1989, the resulting livebirths/retrieval were: Australia 12.5%, the UK 13.0%, the US 15.8%, and 9.9% in Canada. Likewise, guidelines for the regulation of ART centers vary from country to country.

In Canada, there is no regulation nor a mechanism for centralized record-keeping on embryo research. Recently the Canadian Royal Commission on New Reproductive Technologies was asked to make recommendations to the federal government about embryo research. The committee members agreed that any trafficking in human gametes or embryos was unacceptable, and research on the formation of human–animal hybrids, gestation of human zygotes in the uterus of another species, and cloning should be banned.

In Australia, pioneers continued the evolution of the IVF process from natural cycle, which produced Louise Brown, to Clomid, and eventually hMG for controlled ovarian hyperstimulation. To increase the likelihood of success they began to gradually increase the number of embryos transferred to four per cycle.

In 1986, the National Perinatal Statistics Unit published that the perinatal mortality associated with IVF was five times higher than the general population (60 per 1000 vs 12 per 1000). The National Twin Registry, in Melbourne, reported that perinatal mortality from twins was five times higher than singleton pregnancies, and divorce rates in couples who had triplets was three times higher. These results marked the end of the honeymoon for IVF and triggered government legislation. Starting in 1988, the number of embryos for transfer was reduced and by 1993 the perinatal mortality fell to 11 per 1000.

In 1992, 29% of Australian IVF patients and 55% of GIFT patients delivered a live baby after undergoing an average of 3.4 treatment cycles. GIFT is nearly always used when the fallopian tubes are normal; the fallopian tube may contribute to embryo development by removing embryo inhibitory factors or by producing embryo growth factors. The chance of triplets has been lessened by reducing the embryos for transfer to two for IVF and by limiting egg replacement to two for GIFT, when egg quality is optimal.

Currently there are 24 IVF centers in Australia, with 1% of the population attempting an ART procedure. In 1989, Australia accounted for 19% of all ART births throughout the world; 11% of the 1989 ART patients underwent frozen embryo transfer (FET) with a success rate of 13%, which added 1.4% to the overall success rate.

The major factor determining success is the number of cycles attempted, which has increased at Monash University from 2.4 in 1988 to 3.4 in 1991. The Australian government reimburses a global fee for each treatment cycle. The patient pays an additional $400–$1000 depending on whether or not they have private health insurance. Due to reduced cost, nearly twice as many Australians pursue IVF than those in the US.

Controlled ovarian hyperstimulation is usually timed with GnRH agonists and oral contraceptives to avoid nights and weekends, and to allow for batching patients at satellite locations. (Monash University has four satellites 70–180 km from the base hospital.)

Currently, the success rate for FET is 18% per transfer with an average of two embryos transferred. This means that for 11% of women undergoing ART there is a doubling of the overall pregnancy rate from a single stimulation. Pioneering egg maturation for polycystic ovaries patients, the program at Monash University has yielded a fertilization rate of 25%, with an overall success rate of 15%.

In the UK the Warnock Committee convened in 1984 to evaluate and discuss the moral, legal, medical, and political issues of the rapidly evolving reproductive technology.

In 1990, the British Parliament passed the Human Fertilization and Embryology Authority Act (HEFA), which initiated its regulatory role in August, 1991. HEFA licenses clinics for IVF treatment, embryo storage, and research. Since its scope is confined to embryos, GIFT births are not reportable to the agency nor to the public. As a result, there has been a decrease in GIFT procedures in the UK. In 1996, the HEFA published a league table of pregnancy and birth rates, hence causing patients to search for the clinics with the highest rates of birth. This puts pressure on the clinics to transfer the legal maximum of three embryos, which increases the multiple birth rate. In 1996, one third of the 5,542 IVF births in the UK were multiple (two to four babies) as compared to one quarter in 1988.

There are now 120 IVF centers, contributing nearly $1,000,000 in licensing fees to support the HEFA. Despite the presence of the National Health Service (NHS), most British patients pay for their infertility treatment out-of-pocket. Each ART cycle costs about $1,800 in the UK as opposed to an estimated $8,000 in the US.

Besides maintaining a central registry, the HEFA issues a Code of Practice, and proactively evaluates clinical innovations, such as preimplantation genetic diagnosis (PGD) and ICSI. It has compulsory guidelines for embryo research, such as prohibiting cloning by nuclear replacement.

When the HEFA began, the law mandated that cryopreserved embryos be stored for a maximum of five years, unless a formal request for extended storage was received prior to midnight, July 31, 1996. The exact reasoning as to why a five year period was selected was unclear, as the safe storage period appears to be in excess of 50 years. As a result, 3000 healthy embryos were threatened. Attempts were made to extend the storage period until the mother reached the age of 55, which would allow couples longer to decide whether or not to receive their cryopreserved embryos. Unfortunately, the law was not modified and it became each individual clinic's responsibility to contact the parents to receive the formal extension for cryostorage. Since failure to comply with the law could result in clinic license revocation, all facilities holding embryos affected by the storage period did comply. Nearly 3000 embryos were destroyed in the UK on August 1, 1996.

In the United States, there was a major ART scandal. On June 2, 1995, the University of California at Irvine's Center for Reproductive Health was ordered closed due to allegations of medical misconduct by Drs Ricardo Asch, Jose Balmaceda, and Sergio Stone. The charges included prescribing an unapproved infertility drug, concealing over $900,000 in revenue from the university, performing patient research without informed consent, and stealing embryos from younger patients and transferring them to older patients in order to increase the likelihood of success in this difficult population. Published newspaper reports indicated that more than 70 women were affected, with the eggs of one patient allegedly being sent to a zoology laboratory in Wisconsin for research. Since there were no state regulations regarding egg or embryo theft during that time, no state laws were violated. However, prosecutors filed federal mail fraud charges based on mailing false insurance claims. However, prior to federal indictments being issued, Dr Asch fled to Mexico and Dr Balmaceda to Chile. Subsequently, California passed legislation which made it unlawful for anyone to knowingly mishandle gametes and/or embryos. The repercussions include up to five years in jail with a $50,000 fine, as well as possible medical license revocation.

Undoubtedly, the IVF industry has the potential to bring its patients unparalleled happiness or great despair. Public reaction to the allegations about stolen eggs and embryos reflect anger about betrayal by the trusted medical establishment. Many Americans feel the need for greater regulation of privately funded medical procedures, which have operated for a long while in a regulatory vacuum. Despite the fine record of the HEFA in the UK, a central licensing authority may not work for the highly decentralized American system where there are other remedies.

In the US, the Fertility Clinic Success Rate and Certification Act was passed in 1992. The act was only partially implemented due to the failure of the US Department of Health and Human Services to fund it fully. Most centers voluntarily reported their data to the Society of Assisted Reproductive Technology. Recently, the US Centers for Disease Control and Prevention was allocated $1,000,000 to test and upgrade the reporting system and initiate a laboratory certification process. Currently, there are no mandatory guidelines which stipulate how long an IVF center can operate without achieving even one livebirth. For example, in 1994, one third of the centers reporting cryopreservation had never had a livebirth following FET.

In summary, it seems reasonable that each country has a uniform mechanism to report verifiable data to colleagues and patients, with the understanding that success rates may vary with age and diagnosis. Patients should remain confident that gametes and embryos will be handled with respect and in compliance with their informed consent. Efforts should continue to improve success, enhance efficiency, and reduce costs, in order to make this exciting technology accessible to everyone who may benefit from it.

Summary

ART offers the infertile couple another dimension to help achieve their goal of conception, usually after conventional therapy has failed. It is important to balance this exciting modality with the traditional therapies which treat the underlying disease for the patients' ongoing health. Each couple should be thoroughly informed regarding their options by an ethically responsible clinician who places the couple's best interest above their own.

Vaginal ultrasonic-guided ovarian aspiration for IVF

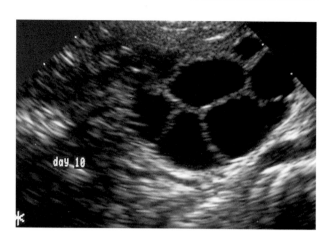

Figure 5.1 Follicular monitoring during controlled ovarian hyperstimulation is accomplished by vaginal ultrasound. Generally, mature follicles are usually greater than 16 mm. When the estradiol exceeds 600 pg/ml and there are at least two mature follicles, usually hCG 10,000 IU is administered and the oocyte retrieval is scheduled 36 hours later.

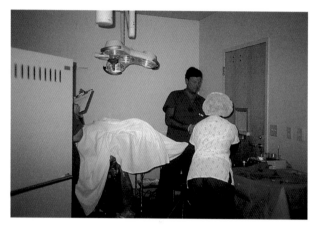

Figure 5.2 For IVF retrieval, IV sedation is administered, using Versed and Fentanyl, in the room adjacent to the egg laboratory. The patient's husband or family member is at the bedside for the vaginal ultrasonic-guided ovarian aspiration.

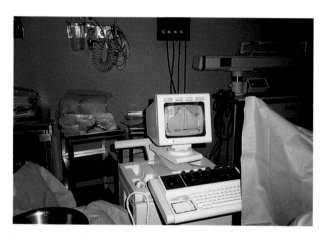

Figure 5.3 The equipment is moved into place for the follicular aspiration.

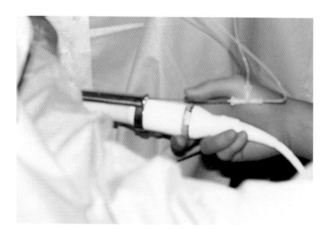

Figure 5.4 The needle guide is used in conjunction with the ultrasound probe to help facilitate follicular cyst aspiration and flushing.

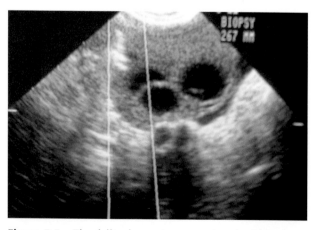

Figure 5.5 The follicular cysts are centered within the biopsy format on the screen.

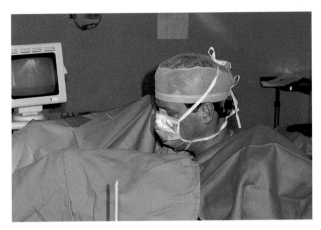

Figure 5.6 Each cyst is systematically visualized, punctured, aspirated, and flushed with tissue culture media.

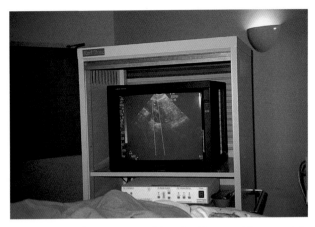

Figure 5.7 The patient and her family are able to watch the procedure on the auxiliary TV screen next to them.

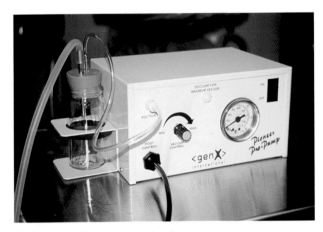

Figure 5.8 The pressure for the system is set at 100 mmHg, with the final flush and aspiration set at 'max' or 400 mmHg.

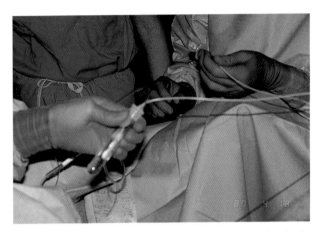

Figure 5.9 The follicular fluid is collected in individual test tubes.

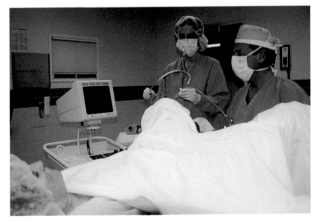

Figure 5.10 The scrub nurse monitors the volume of fluid in each test tube, changing to a new one when nearly full.

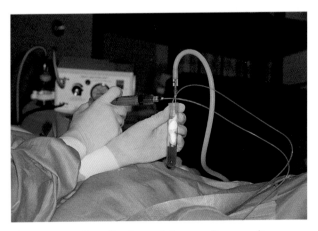

Figure 5.11 Usually, 2 cc of tissue culture media are flushed when the cyst is completely collapsed. This helps dislodge any remaining oocytes.

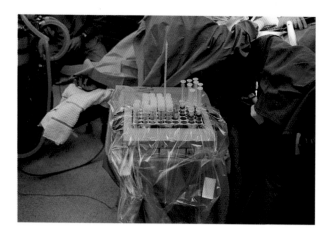

Figure 5.12   Each test tube is set in a warmer to keep the temperature constant.

Gamete identification and preparation

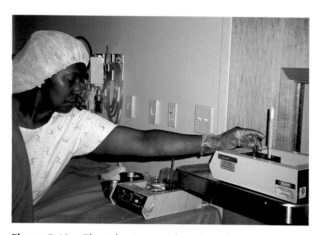

Figure 5.13   The tube is passed to the adjacent egg laboratory.

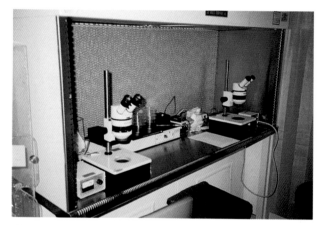

Figure 5.14   Inside the IVF laboratory, a hood limits contaminants in the air.

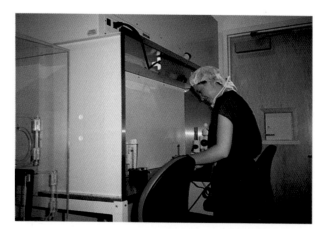

Figure 5.15   The biologist takes each test tube containing follicular fluid and aspirate to the hood.

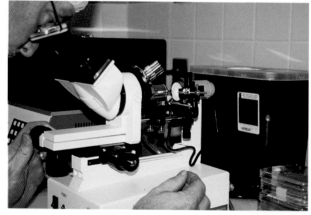

Figure 5.16   The fluid is placed into a Petri dish and scanned.

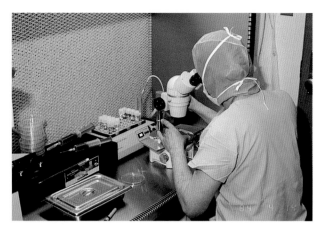

Figure 5.17   Each oocyte is taken from the follicular fluid and placed into another Petri dish with tissue culture media.

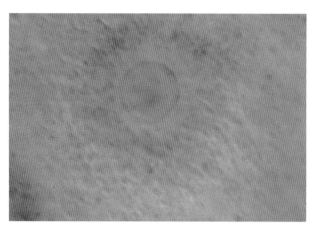

Figure 5.18   The oocytes are graded for quality, ideally looking for mature oocytes.

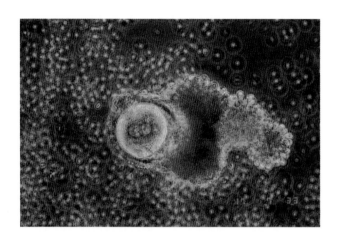

Figure 5.19   Processed spermatozoa are placed into the Petri dish in order to inseminate the oocyte.

Fertilization and embryonic division

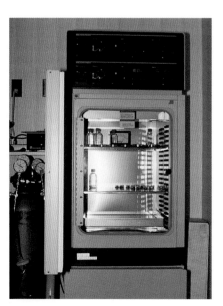

Figure 5.20
The Petri dish containing the gametes is placed into an incubator to enable fertilization.

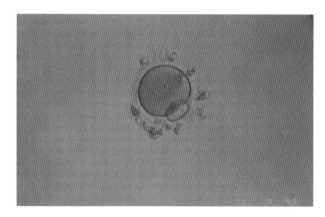

Figure 5.21   Each Petri dish containing the gametes is checked for fertilization, which activates the oocyte by increasing metabolic activity. The haploid egg nucleus and the haploid sperm nucleus become the female and male pronuclei.

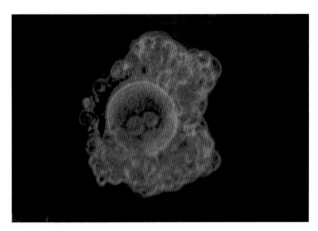

Figure 5.22 A zygote is formed from a normally fertilized oocyte with two pronuclei and two polar bodies seen. Both pronuclei enter a phase of DNA synthesis with chromosome replication arranged on a common spindle.

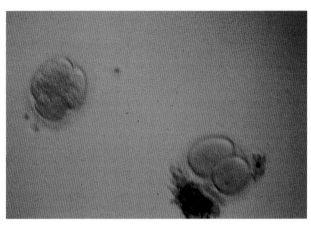

Figure 5.23 The rapidity of cellular division varies with each embryo, as seen with these embryos, one two cell and one four cell; both were fertilized at the same time. The two-cell stage is derived from the first cell division. Cleavage into the four- and eight-cell stages are due to cytoplasmic furrows of clefts which produce blastomeres.

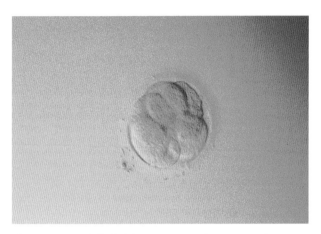

Figure 5.24 Cell divisions are asynchronous and may produce odd numbered embryos, as seen in this five-cell embryo. At this point the morula is surrounded by the zona pellucida and thus is the same size as the original unfertilized oocyte.

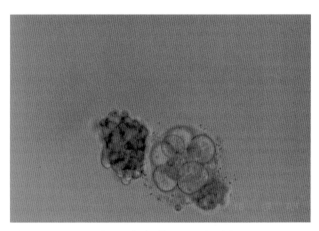

Figure 5.25 At the eight-cell stage, the blastomeres form junctional complexes and gain an epithelial character called compaction.

Day 3 embryo transfer

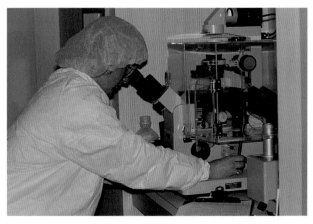

Figure 5.26 The embryos are scanned and graded prior to transfer, which is usually planned for 72 hours after oocyte retrieval.

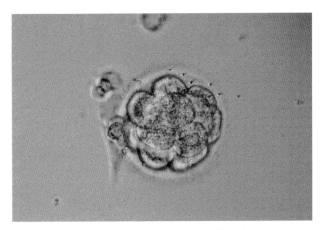

Figure 5.27 The symmetry of each cell and amount of fragmentation are assessed. Most of the inherent cumulus has been lost, as seen in this embryo prior to transfer.

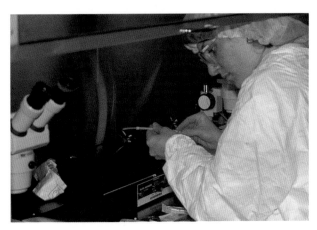

Figure 5.28 All the embryos for transfer are placed into one Petri dish prior to loading the Wallace catheter.

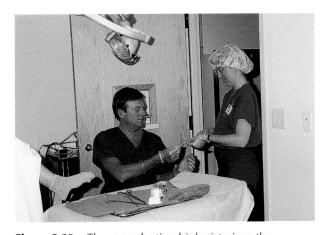

Figure 5.29 The reproductive biologist gives the catheter containing the embryos to the author for embryo transfer.

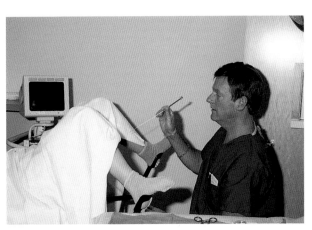

Figure 5.30 The cervix is wiped with tissue culture media, the cervical mucus vigorously lavaged, and the dummy trial transfer Wallace catheter is placed into the uterus under abdominal ultrasound monitoring. The actual Wallace catheter is loaded, and passed into the uterus taking care not to contact the vaginal walls. When approximately 1 cm from the fundus, the embryos are very gently placed into the uterine cavity. The catheter is checked to be sure that all the embryos have been released into the uterine cavity, thus completing the embryo transfer.

Laparoscopic ovarian aspiration for GIFT

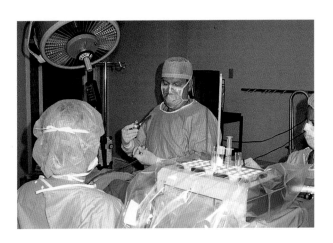

Figure 5.31 For GIFT, the operating room is used with a general anesthetic administered.

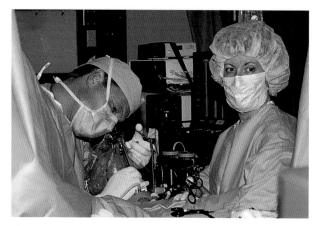

Figure 5.32 Laparoscopic visualization of the pelvic organs is accomplished using CO_2 gas for peritoneal distention.

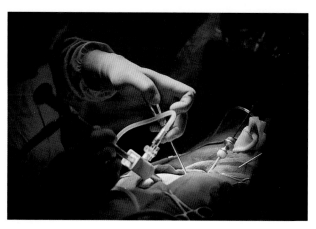

Figure 5.33 The trocars are placed to facilitate oocyte aspiration.

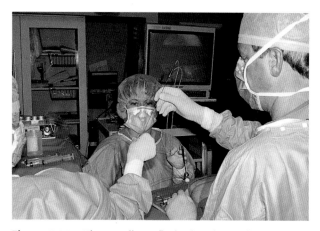

Figure 5.34 The needle is flushed and introduced into the abdominal cavity.

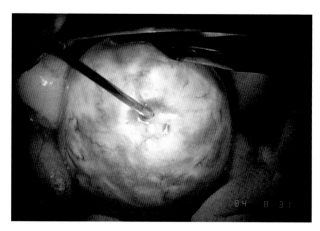

Figure 5.35 Each follicle is aspirated systematically.

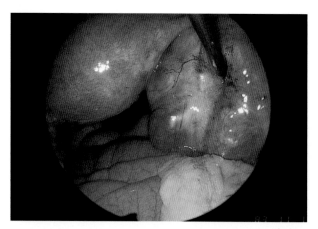

Figure 5.36 Often, it is necessary to pass the needle through one follicle in order to reach the deeper follicles.

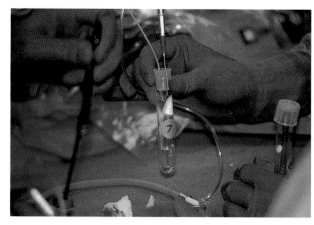

Figure 5.37 The follicular fluid is collected in test tubes.

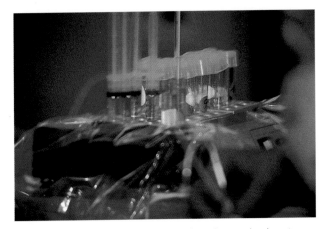

Figure 5.38 The test tubes are placed into the heating block to keep the temperature constant.

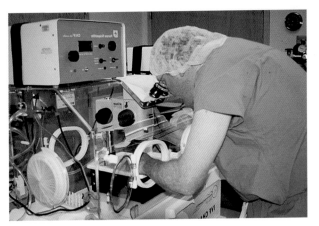

Figure 5.39 The aspirated fluid is scanned in the laboratory for oocytes.

Transtubal transfer

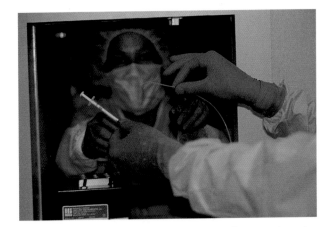

Figure 5.40 When all the oocytes have been retrieved, usually three to four oocytes, with an aliquot of processed spermatozoa, are placed into the gamete transfer catheter and handed to the physician.

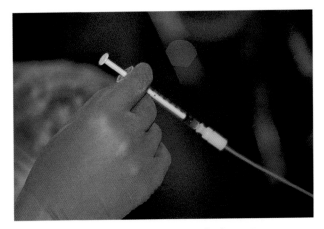

Figure 5.41 The scrub nurse controls the syringe.

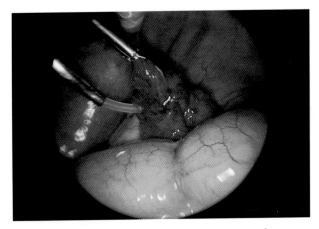

Figure 5.42 The catheter is placed approximately 3 cm into the distal fallopian tube.

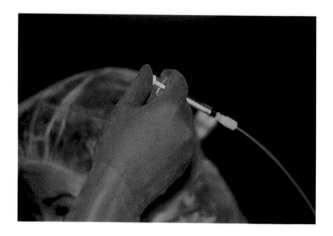

Figure 5.43 When the plunger is depressed, expressing the gametes, the catheter is slowly withdrawn and checked to confirm discharge of all oocytes and spermatozoa.

Micromanipulation – work station

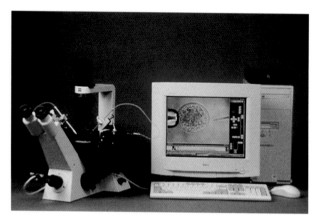

Figure 5.44 If micromanipulation is planned, as part of an IVF cycle to assist fertilization (ICSI) or implantation (assisted hatching), this is accomplished at the IVF work station (courtesy of Jerome Conia, Ph.D., Cell Robotics, Inc.).

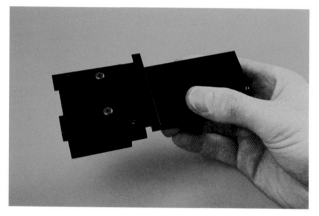

Figure 5.45 The 1480 nm laser module couples the diode laser to the microscope optics (courtesy of Jerome Conia, Ph.D., Cell Robotics, Inc.).

Laser-assisted hatching

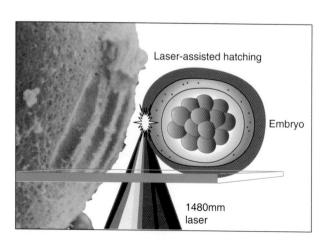

Laser-assisted hatching

Embryo

1480mm laser

Figure 5.46 Use of the laser for assisted hatching is currently being investigated. It appears that this technique is more accurate, reproducible, and easily learned than the microinjection of acid tyrode solution currently used. It can be more easily performed, monitored, and repeated consistently in multiple locations on the same embryo. The 1480 nm diode laser is a small near-infrared laser with a small collimated lens that may be inserted into the inverted microscope. The laser energy is absorbed by the zona pellucida but not by the water contained in the tissue culture media. A shallow trench is made into the zona pellucida tangentially (courtesy of Jerome Conia, Ph.D., Cell Robotics, Inc.).

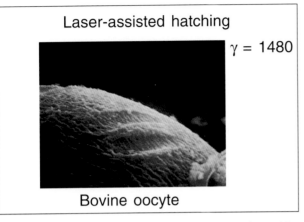

Figure 5.47 Multiple practice trenches are made in this bovine oocyte (courtesy of Jerome Conia, Ph.D., Cell Robotics, Inc.).

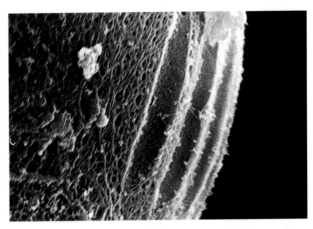

Figure 5.48 A close-up of the precise multiple trenches is seen, showing the laser precision and control of depth (courtesy of Jerome Conia, Ph.D., Cell Robotics, Inc.).

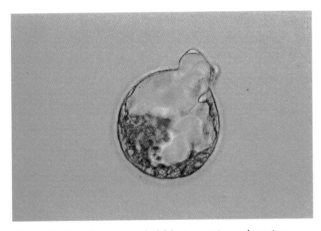

Figure 5.49 This expanded blastocyst is undergoing early embryonic hatching, which occurs in vivo prior to attaching to the uterine epithelium. As further absorption of fluid occurs, the hatched blastocyst swells to a diameter of 0.25 mm.

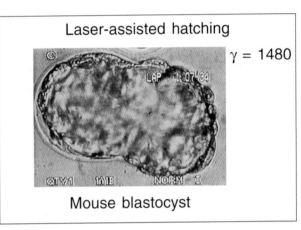

Figure 5.50 A hatching mouse blastocyst is seen after laser-assisted hatching has been completed (courtesy of Mitchel Schiewe, Ph.D., HCLD).

ICSI

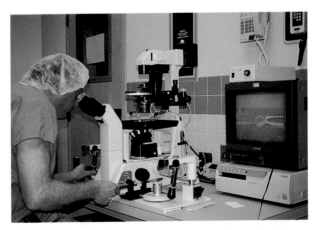

Figure 5.51 Micromanipulation has revolutionized the treatment of male factor infertility due to oligospermia by using ICSI.

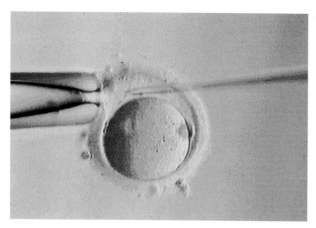

Figure 5.52 Subzonal sperm injection (SUZI) was initially recommended until ICSI became more widely utilized for IVF treatment of male factor infertility (courtesy of Jerome Conia, Ph.D., Cell Robotics, Inc.).

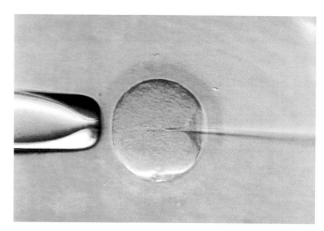

Figure 5.53 For ICSI, a single sperm is selected and the zona is punctured. Orientation of the polar body during the procedure is critical to minimize chromosome damage (courtesy of Mitchel Schiewe, Ph.D., HCLD).

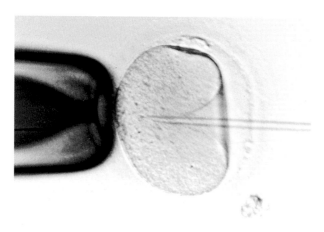

Figure 5.54 The ooplasm is further invaginated until the sperm may be injected (courtesy of Mitchel Schiewe, Ph.D., HCLD).

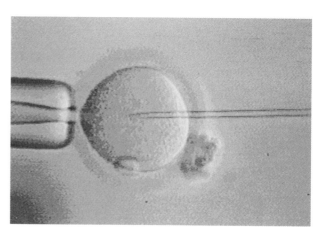

Figure 5.55 After the sperm is injected into the cytoplasm, the glass pipette is withdrawn (courtesy of Mitchel Schiewe, Ph.D., HCLD).

Embryo cryopreservation

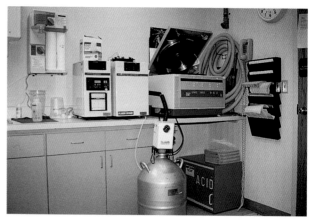

Figure 5.56 For cryopreservation of remaining embryos, a Planer freezer is used to gradually cool the zygotes.

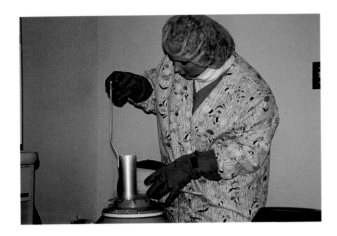

Figure 5.57 The cryopreserved embryos are placed into liquid nitrogen. The first successful pregnancy following transfer of a frozen embryo was reported in 1983, by Alan Trounson, Ph.D., at Monash University in Melbourne, Australia.

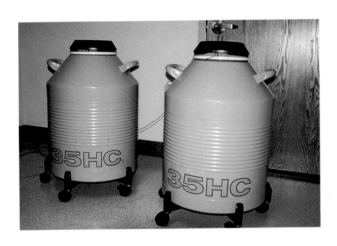

Figure 5.58 The embryos may remain frozen in storage until transfer is elected by the couple.

Day 5 blastocyst transfer

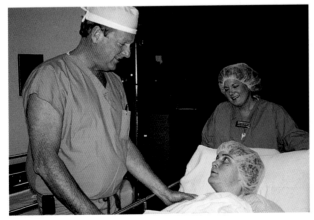

Figure 5.59 Prior to embryo transfer, the patient is greeted by the author and the IVF nurse coordinator.

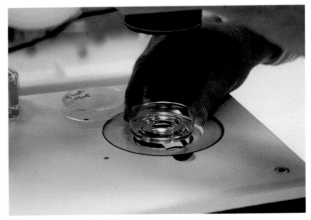

Figure 5.60 The embryologist assesses the growth of the embryo prior to transfer.

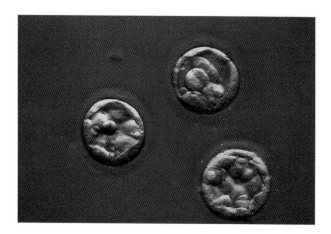

Figure 5.61 The blastocyst cavity begins to form when the cell number reaches between 32 and 58, as seen in these early blastocysts. The blastomeres rearrange into an inner cell mass situated internally, surrounded by an outer trophoblast layer of cells. These trophoblast cells form a tight epithelial layer which secretes fluid into the blastocyst cavity.

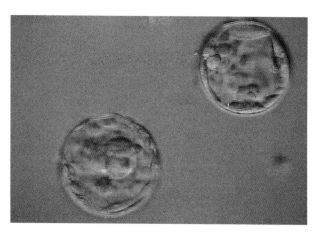

Figure 5.62 This slide depicts an expanded blastocyst which occurs as the fluid accumulates in the blastocyst cavity.

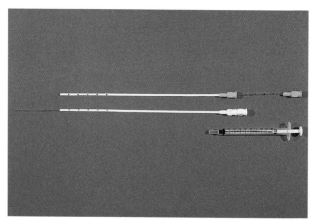

Figure 5.63 McNamee has described an improved technique for embryo transfer using a Wallace catheter. The cervical mucus is irrigated with tissue culture media using a flexible tip, such as an Angiocath.

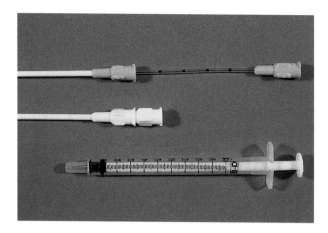

Figure 5.64 A solid Edwards–Wallace catheter, 23 cm, is then passed transcervically to insure easy access. (The preceding month prior to transfer, the uterine depth and canal location had been recorded at the time of uterine sounding and sonohysterogram to exclude intra-uterine pathology.)

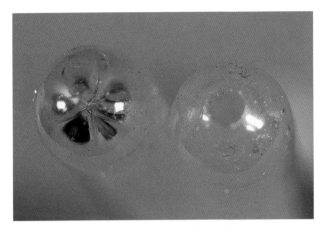

Figure 5.65 A close-up of the solid and open Edwards–Wallace catheters show the soft beveled tips which facilitate passing them through the cervix atraumatically.

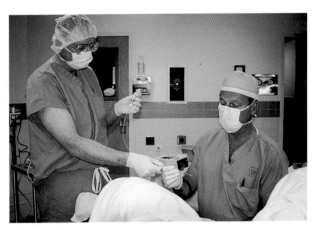

Figure 5.66 The embryologist hands the loaded transfer catheter to the author for intra-uterine placement.

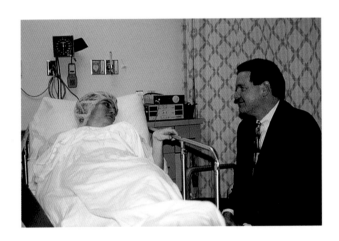

Figure 5.67 The patient is reunited with her family for a short time following embryo transfer. She is usually discharged home about an hour later to resume her normal activities.

OHSS

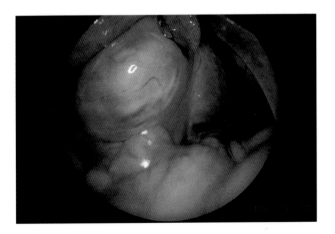

Figure 5.68 OHSS seen with moderately enlarged ovaries in this patient undergoing laparoscopy to exclude ectopic pregnancy following GIFT conception.

BIBLIOGRAPHY

Al-Shawaf T, Harper D, Linehan J, et al: Transfer of embryos into the uterus: How much do technical factors affect pregnancy rates? *J Assist Reprod Gen* **10**:31–9, 1993.

Annas G: The shadowlands-secrets, lies, and assisted reproduction. *N Engl J Med* **339**:935–9, 1998.

Atri M, Tran C, Bret P: Accuracy of endovaginal sonography for the detection of fallopian tube blockage. *J Ultrasound Med* **13**:429–34, 1994.

Baird P: Human embryo research in Canada: legal and policy aspects. *Hum Reprod* **12**:2343–5, 1997.

Bassil S, Godin P, Stallaert S, et al: Ovarian hyperstimulation syndrome: a review. *Assist Reprod Rev* **5**:90–6, 1995.

Beerendonk C, van Dop P, Merkus J: Ovarian hyperstimulation syndrome: facts and fallacies. *Obstet Gynecol Surv* **53**:439–49, 1998.

Belaisch-Allart J, De Mouzon J, Lapousterie C, et al: The effect of hCG supplementation after combined GnRH agonist/hMG treatment in an IVF program. *Hum Reprod* **5**:163–70, 1990.

Blazar A, Hogan J, Seifer D, et al: The impact of hydrosalpinx on successful pregnancy in tubal factor infertility treated by in vitro fertilization. *Fertil Steril* **67**:517–20, 1997.

Byers K: Infertility and in vitro fertilization. *J Legal Med* **18**:265–313, 1997.

Centers for Disease Control and Prevention, American Society for Reproductive Medicine, Resolve: 1995 Assisted Reproductive Technology Success Rates, December, 1997.

Centers for Disease Control and Prevention: 1996 Data on Births in the United States, February, 1999.

Chung P, Yeko T, Mayer J, et al: Gamete intrafallopian transfer. Does smoking play a role? *J Reprod Med* **42**:65–70, 1997.

Craft I, Al-Shawaf T: IVF versus GIFT. *J Assist Reprod Gen* **9**:424–6, 1992.

Dickson D: Reducing embryo implants in IVF. *Nature Med* **3**:1309, 1997.

Drews U: *Color Atlas of Embryology*. New York, Thieme Medical Publishers, 1995.

Edwards R, Beard H: Destruction of cryopreserved embryos: UK law dictated the destruction of 3000 cryopreserved human embryos. *Hum Reprod* **12**:3–5, 1997.

Egbase P, Sharhan M, Othman S, et al: Incidence of microbial growth from the tip of the embryo transfer catheter after embryo transfer in relation to clinical pregnancy rate following in vitro fertilization and embryo transfer. *Hum Reprod* **11**:687–9, 1996.

Gardner D, Vella P, Lane M, et al: Culture and transfer of human blastocysts increases implantation rates and reduces the need for multiple embryo transfers. *Fertil Steril* **69**:84–8, 1998.

Gonen Y, Jacobson W, Casper R: Gonadotropin suppression with oral contraceptives before in vitro fertilization. *Fertil Steril* **53**:282–91, 1990.

Gray C: High-tech conceptions: Can Canada afford them? *CMAJ* **138**:948–9, 1988.

Guzick DS, Yao YA, Berga SL, et al: Endometriosis impairs the efficacy of gamete intrafallopian transfer: results of a case-control study. *Fertil Steril* **62**:1186–91, 1994.

Guzick DS, Carson SA, Coutifaris C, et al: Efficacy of superovulation and intrauterine insemination in the treatment of infertility. National Cooperative Reproductive Medicine Network. *N Engl J Med* **340**:177–83, 1999.

Hughes E, Yeo J, Claman P, et al: Cigarette smoking and the outcomes of in vitro fertilization: measurement of effect size and levels of action. *Fertil Steril* **62**:807–12, 1994.

Johnson M: Genetic risks of intracytoplasmic sperm injection in the treatment of male infertility: recommendations for genetic counseling and screening. *Fertil Steril* **70**:397–411, 1998.

Johnston I: Some Australian perspectives on in-vitro fertilization. *Hum Reprod* **11**:25–31, 1996.

Jones H: The time has come. *Fertil Steril* **65**:1090–2, 1996.

Kim A, McKay H, Keltz M, et al: Sonohysterographic screening before in vitro fertilization. *Fertil Steril* **69**:841–4, 1998.

Lancaster P: International comparisons of Assisted Reproduction. *Asst Reprod Rev* **2**:212–21, 1992.

La Sala G, Montanari R, Dessanti L, et al: The role of diagnostic hysteroscopy and endometrial biopsy in assisted reproductive technologies. *Fertil Steril* **70**:378–80, 1998.

Lawler A, Gearhart J: Genetic counseling for patients who will be undergoing treatment with assisted reproductive technology. *Fertil Steril* **70**:412–13, 1998.

Legro R, Shacklefor D, Moessner J, et al: ART in women 40 and over: Is the cost worth it? *J Reprod Med* **42**:76–82, 1997.

Liu H-C, Cohen J, Alikani M, et al: Assisted hatching facilitates earlier implantation. *Fertil Steril* **60**:871–5, 1993.

Mansour R, Aboulghar M, Serour G: Dummy embryo transfer: a technique that minimizes the problems of embryo transfer and improves the pregnancy rate in human in vitro fertilization. *Fertil Steril* **54**:578–81, 1990.

Martin P, Welch H: Probabilities for singleton and multiple pregnancies after in vitro fertilization. *Fertil Steril* **70**:478–81, 1998.

McLaughlin D, Troike D, Tegenkamp T, McCarthy D: Tubal ovum transfer: a Catholic-approved alternative to in vitro fertilization. *Lancet* **1**:214–15, 1987.

Meldrum D: GnRH agonists as adjuncts for in vitro fertilization. *Obstet Gynecol Surg* **44**:314–22, 1989.

Meldrum D, Gardner D: Two-embryo transfer—the future looks bright. *N Engl J Med* **339**:624–5, 1998.

Meyer W, Beyler S: Deleterious effects of hydrosalpinges on in vitro fertilization and endometrial integrin expression. *Assist Reprod Rev* **5**:201–3, 1995.

Pearlstone A, Fournet N, Gambone J, et al: Ovulation induction in woman age 40 and older: the importance of basal follicle-stimulating hormone level and chronological age. *Fertil Steril* **58**: 674–9, 1992.

Perone N: In vitro fertilization and embryo transfer: a historical perspective. *J Reprod Med* **39**:695–700, 1994.

Poindexter A, Thompson D, Gibbons W, et al: Residual embryos in failed embryo transfer. *Fertil Steril* **46**:262–7, 1986.

Roest J, van Heusden A, Mous H, et al: The ovarian response as a predictor for successful in vitro fertilization treatment after the age of 40 years. *Fertil Steril* **66**:969–73, 1996.

Scher G, Zouves C, Feinman M, et al: Prolonged coasting: an effective method for preventing severe ovarian hyperstimulation syndrome in patients undergoing in vitro fertilization. *Hum Reprod* **10**:3107–22, 1995.

Scholtes M, Zeilmaker G: A prospective, randomized study of embryo transfer results after 3 or 5 days of embryo culture in in vitro fertilization. *Fertil Steril* **65**:1245–8, 1996.

Schoolcraft W, Schlenker T, Gee M, et al: Assisted hatching in the treatment of poor prognosis in vitro fertilization candidates. *Fertil Steril* **62**:551–4, 1994.

Schoolcraft W, Schlenker T, Gee M, et al: Improved controlled ovarian hyperstimulation in poor responder in vitro fertilization patients with a microdose follicle-stimulating hormone flare, growth hormone protocol. *Fertil Steril* **67**:93–7, 1997.

Schutze K, Clement-Sengewald A, Ashkin A: Zona drilling and sperm insertion with combined laser microbeam and optical tweezers. *Fertil Steril* **61**:783–6, 1994.

Scott R, Navot D: Enhancement of ovarian responsiveness with microdoses of gonadotropin-releasing hormone agonist during ovulation induction for in vitro fertilization. *Fertil Steril* **61**:880–97, 1994.

Sharif K, Afnan M, Lenton W, et al: Do patients need to remain in bed following embryo transfer? The Birmingham experience of 103 in-vitro fertilization cycles with no bed rest following embryo transfer. *Hum Reprod* **10**:1427–31, 1995.

Smitz J, Devroey P, Faguer B, et al: A prospective randomized comparison of intramuscular or intravaginal natural progesterone as a luteal phase and early pregnancy supplement. *Hum Reprod* **7**:168–79, 1992.

Stolwijk A, Zielhuis G, Sauer M, et al: The impact of the woman's age on the success of standard and donor in vitro fertilization. *Fertil Steril* **67**:702–10, 1997.

Strohmer H, Feichtinger W: Successful clinical application of laser for micromanipulation in an in vitro fertilization program. *Fertil Steril* **58**:212–14, 1992.

Tadir Y, Neev J, Berns M: Laser in assisted reproduction and genetics. *J Assist Reprod Gen* **9**:303–5, 1992.

Templeton A, Morris J: Reducing the risk of multiple births by transfer of two embryos after in vitro fertilization. *N Engl J Med* **339**:573–7, 1998.

Trounson A, Wood C: IVF and related technology. *Med J Aust* **158**:853–7, 1993.

UCLA Syllabus: 11th Annual In Vitro Fertilization and Embryo Transfer Comprehensive Update. Santa Barbara, CA, July 19–22, 1998.

Vandromme J, Chasse E, Lejeune B, et al: Hydrosalpinges in in-vitro fertilization: an unfavorable feature. *Hum Reprod* **10**:576–81, 1995.

Velde E, Cohlen B: The management of infertility. *N Engl J Med* **340**:224–6, 1999.

Vrtovec H, Tomazevic T: Preventing severe ovarian hyperstimulation syndrome in an in vitro fertilization/embryo transfer program. *J Reprod Med* **40**:37–40, 1995.

White G: Choices: Biomedical ethics and women's health – Crisis in assisted conception: the British approach to an American Dilemma. *J Wom Health* **7**:321–8, 1998.

Wilkins-Haug L, Rein M, Hornstein M: Oligospermic men: the role of karyotype analysis prior to intracytoplasmic sperm injection. *Fertil Steril* **67**:612–14, 1997.

Yee B, Rosen G, Chacon R, et al: Gamete intrafallopian transfer: the effect of the number of eggs used and the depth of gamete placement on pregnancy initiation. *Fertil Steril* **52**:639–44, 1989.

Yovich J, Edirisinghe W, Cummings J: Evaluation of luteal support therapy in a randomized controlled study within a gamete intrafallopian transfer program. *Fertil Steril* **55**:131–9, 1991.

Zeyneloglu H, Arici A, Olive D: Adverse effects of hydrosalpinx on pregnancy rates after in vitro fertilization – embryo transfer. *Fertil Steril* **70**:492–9, 1998.

6 Conclusion

Putting it all together, after analyzing the conflicting data available in the literature, seems to be a monumental task. A logical, common-sense approach to current indications for each procedure is desirable. Several questions need to be answered when integrating these new technologies:

(1) What are the safety considerations regarding hysteroscopic laser/rollerball surgery?
(2) Is it prudent to remove ovarian cysts through the laparoscope?
(3) How predictive is CA-125 for ovarian malignancy?
(4) Is operative laparoscopy better than laparotomy?
(5) Is laparoscopic assisted vaginal hysterectomy (LAVH) better?
(6) What is the chance of adhesion formation following conservative pelvic surgery?
(7) What is the future for tubal surgery?
(8) When should assisted reproductive technology (ART) be considered?
(9) What are the ethical implications of shared-risk (refund) programs in ART?

Safety considerations – operative hysteroscopy

Five cases of fatal and one case of near-fatal gas embolus have been described following the hysteroscopic use of gas-cooled coaxial Nd:YAG laser fibers. Cardiovascular collapse, cardiac arrest, and death in the majority of cases occurred from massive air absorption into the venous vasculature and heart. Inappropriate use of sheathed fibers, cooled by air, nitrogen, or CO_2, at 200–2000 ml per minute was responsible for the surgical mishaps. Only a fluid medium should be used for operative hysteroscopy, with a bare or drawn-contact fiber, when using the Nd:YAG laser.

One case of small bowel injury has been reported following a rollerball endometrial ablation. The patient presented two days following her endoscopic procedure with an acute abdomen. Subsequent bowel repair and hysterectomy failed to demonstrate uterine perforation; an area of thermal injury was noted through the uterine wall to the serosa, after using 40 watts of electrical coagulation. This is quite disconcerting as similar injuries may become more apparent as the number of these procedures are performed, just as in the case of bowel burn following laparoscopic tubal fulgeration with unipolar cautery in the early 1970s. Care should be taken to move the rollerball continuously when activating the electrical current. Endometrial ablation with Gynecare's Thermachoice uterine balloon therapy should drastically reduce the complications inherent in earlier endometrial ablative therapies.

Laparoscopic removal of ovarian cysts

Forty-two cases of ovarian neoplasms managed by laparoscopy and subsequently found to be malignant were reported in a survey of members of the Society of Gynecological Oncologists. The cases were managed nearly equally, by aspiration, partial excision, and complete excision. 'Benign characteristics' were noted in:

81% unilateral
67% < 8 cm
62% cystic
48% unilocular
31% all four characteristics
24% three of four characteristics

Subsequent laparotomy occurred:

17% at the time of laparoscopy
71% following laparoscopy (average interval 5 weeks)
12% none

At least half the patients had stage II–IV disease. The conclusions reached were:

(1) Attempted laparoscopic management of benign-appearing ovarian cancers is not uncommon.
(2) Attempts at partial or complete excision through the laparoscope are common, along with delays in subsequent definitive surgery.
(3) Strict guidelines for optimal patient care should be developed after careful evaluation of this procedure.

This raises the question whether benign-appearing masses should be evaluated and managed by laparoscopy? The incidence of cancer in benign-appearing pelvic masses varies by age group:

< 2% under age 30
7–11% ages 30–50
8% over age 50

The clinical reluctance to manage adnexal masses by laparoscopy includes:

(1) the risk of spillage of a malignant cyst
(2) spillage of a mucinous tumor
(3) spillage of a dermoid cyst

It has been reported that spillage of a malignant or mucinous cyst has no effect on prognosis. The factors which predict tumor recurrence are:

(1) tumor differentiation
(2) dense adhesions
(3) ascites > 250 cc

There appears to be no prognostic value determined by:

(1) bilaterality
(2) cyst rupture
(3) capsule penetration
(4) tumor size
(5) histologic subtype
(6) patient age
(7) year of diagnosis
(8) post-operative treatment

The five-year survival rate was reported to be 98% for those patients without dense adhesions and large-volume ascites. Nine patients with dermoid tumors managed by laparoscopy were reported. Three patients who had tumor spillage underwent second-look laparoscopy, with no de novo adhesions found. Thus, the risk of spillage of a malignant, mucinous, or dermoid cyst appears to have no long-term effects on potential outcome.

Ca-125

Ca-125 is a tumor marker for epithelial cancer. It is reported to be positive in 80% of the serum in women with ovarian malignancy. The level increases as the disease progresses, but mostly in non-mucinous ovarian cancers. It is falsely elevated in women with:

(1) pelvic inflammatory disease (PID)
(2) endometriosis
(3) fibroids
(4) pregnancy
(5) ovarian hyperstimulation syndrome

Its predictive value varies with age:

(1) 36% accuracy in pre-menopausal females
(2) 87% accuracy in post-menopausal females

Its usefulness increases when used in conjunction with ultrasound and pelvic examination.

Operative laparoscopy versus laparotomy

Reproductive success should be used to evaluate the results of conservative surgery for endometriosis in infertile females. However, no sufficient data in controlled series exist to objectively compare results of patients with endometriosis treated by laparoscopy or laparotomy. This is even more apparent when evaluating morbidity, pain relief, and occurrence. Laparotomy facilitates the surgeon's ability to:

(1) remove the lesion entirely
(2) lyse adhesions
(3) restore anatomy
(4) reperitonealize
(5) suture
(6) operate more rapidly

There appears to be equal success whether an operating microscope, loupes, or the naked eye is used with electrocautery or the CO_2 laser. A uterine suspension may be helpful to reduce adhesion formation along with Interceed or Seprafilm. No apparent reduction of adhesions is noted if heparin, antihistamines, steroids, or Hyskon is used. In 600 patients, the success rate is reported as 38%.

Laparoscopic treatment of endometriosis is primarily beneficial to reduce the patient's recuperative time. The lesions may be resected, excised, ablated, vaporized, or coagulated with the laser or electrocautery with each technique being equally effective. Since laparoscopic suturing is difficult, reperitonealization and closure of the ovary after cyst removal is usually not done. The reported success rate is 48%.

Indications for operative laparoscopy need to be refined by well-controlled multicenter randomized studies comparing laparoscopy to laparotomy.

Is LAVH better?

Since 1989, when LAVH was first described, there has been a dramatic increase in the number of procedures performed. LAVH is a spectrum of procedures to reduce the usual cost and morbidity of total abdominal hysterectomy (TAH). However, it remains controversial, as advocates state that TAH can be converted into LAVH, saving money and convalescent time, and critics contend that LAVH takes longer to perform and is more expensive. Currently, about 70% of all hysterectomies performed in the United States are through an abdominal incision. By the year 2000, estimates are that more than half of the abdominal surgeries will be performed laparoscopically. It is difficult to compare efficacy (outcomes when the procedure is performed by an expert, usually published in the literature) versus efficiency (outcomes when performed by an average practitioner) when evaluating the place of LAVH. In comparative published studies, the complication rate for LAVH was similar to TAH (8% vs 8.7%), but major complications (urinary tract, bowel, vascular injury, etc.) were more common (2.6% vs 0.9%). It is probable that the use of endoscopic staplers, applied to the uterine arteries, is responsible for the disproportionate number of ureteral injuries. It appears that inadequate training and inexperience contribute to the gap between efficacy, by the experts, and efficiency, as experienced by the average practising physician. The complication rate following vaginal hysterectomy (VH) was 6.8%.

When comparing the operating times published in the world's literature, LAVH averaged 117 minutes, TAH 104 minutes, and VH 125 minutes. The length of time varied based on the surgeons' experience and skill, as well as the amount of laparoscopic dissection performed prior to completing the procedure vaginally. One inexperienced group from Northwestern averaged 4 hours. Of those surgeons, 29 had performed an average of three LAVHs, 13 did one, and 4 had performed more than five. Concomitantly, the cost for LAVH in this group was $3604 higher than for TAH. In a Deloitte & Touche study, the most experienced group showed a decrease in cost for LAVH vs TAH, largely in part

due to the decreased length of stay (1.5 days). The indirect convalescent cost saving is more difficult to measure. The average return to work for LAVH patients is 3–4 weeks as opposed to 5–6 weeks following TAH. The advantage of this procedure for the self-employed and for those without disability payments is obvious.

It seems reasonable that LAVH performed on the appropriately selected patient, by a skilled surgeon with the correct equipment, should be able to reduce overall cost and morbidity, with a reduction in postoperative pain and cosmetic trauma, with a more rapid return to work. Unfortunately, many residency programs in the United States do not provide the training required to become skilled laparoscopists and vaginal surgeons. This may be due to a combination of declining case volume as well as the market demand for excellence. Suboptimal clinical outcomes will most likely follow those surgeons who have not obtained an adequate degree of training or skill. A possible solution is the completion of a Reproductive Surgery Fellowship, after the completion of an OB-GYN residency or Reproductive Endocrinology fellowship. This one year fellowship is offered through the American Society for Reproductive Surgery and Medicine; the author has qualified as a preceptor for those who may be interested. The experience should help the preceptee gain skills and confidence when performing this procedure. LAVH skill obtained will help prevent the dilemma of being unable to perform the intended removal of the ovaries at the time of VH, which has been reported to be about a third of the time.

Adhesion formation

After reproductive surgery, adhesion reformation has been reported to be as high as 85% with de novo formation 51%. Fibrosis of unlysed fibrin begin three days after serosal trauma and is complete by 21 days. Adhesions can adversely affect patients by causing infertility, pain, bowel obstruction, and complicating subsequent surgery.

The surgeon is the single most important factor in preventing subsequent adhesion formation by gentle tissue handling, insisting upon meticulous hemostasis, minimizing ischemia and tissue trauma, and by selecting the proper suture for the correct indication. Research has concentrated on developing effective surgical adjuvants to reduce subsequent adhesions by:

• reducing or preventing peritoneal trauma
• preventing the serous exudate coagulation

- eliminating fibrin from the surgical field
- separating fibrin-coated peritoneal surfaces until mesothelization has occurred (usually 5–7 days)
- limiting fibroblastic activity once it has begun

Current barrier methods to reduce the chance for adhesion reformation include: Gore-Tex®, Interceed, and Seprafilm. Gore-Tex® is a thin sheet of poly-tetrafluoroethylene with a micropore architecture (< 1 micron diameter) which prevents cellular invasion during the healing process. It is an inert, non-absorbable membrane which should be sutured in situ with small permanent sutures. If subsequent removal is desired, usually this can be accomplished laparoscopically. Three clinical trials, involving 77 patients, demonstrated reduction in subsequent adhesions. Interceed, or TC7, is composed of oxidized regenerated cellulose, which becomes a gel within 8 hours, and forms a gelatinous cocoon around the tissue within 20 hours. It is a pliable, woven material, which is amenable for laparoscopic placement, followed by irrigation by heparinized Ringers lactate. Its disadvantage is that it becomes ineffective when in contact with blood, which causes Interceed to turn black (if this occurs, it should be removed). It has been evaluated by nine clinical trials in 450 patients, and has been shown to be effective. The newest absorbable adjunct, Seprafilm, is composed of a chemically modified hyaluronic acid with carboxymethylcellulose. It acts as a barrier between two traumatized peritoneal surfaces and is absorbed within 7 days. Two clinical trials, involving 310 patients, showed a reduction in the incidence, extent, and amount of subsequent adhesions.

Early second-look laparoscopy (< 6 weeks post-operatively) is helpful to evaluate healing following reproductive surgery as well as to lyse filmy adhesions. Late-interval second-look laparoscopy (one year) is ineffective. It has been demonstrated by third-look laparoscopy that 50% of adhesions lysed by early second-look laparoscopy did not return. A multicenter study reported the incidence of adhesions following operative laparoscopy as evaluated by early second-look laparoscopy to be:

67% reformation
16% de novo adhesions

The incidence of adhesion reformation with operative laparoscopy was similar to those following laparotomy, but de novo adhesions were less. However, there was no clear-cut effect on pregnancy rates by lysing adhesions at early second-look laparoscopy.

In laparotomies, comparing lasers versus electrocautery, the rate of recurrence was less likely in the laser group. For neosalpingostomy by laparotomy, the pregnancy rates for the laser and electrosurgical groups were similar (53% vs 52%), but the time to conception was shortened (10 months vs 13 months). In evaluating laser laparoscopic treatment of endometriosis by early second-look laparoscopy, one study reported no de novo adhesions with a reduction of peritoneal and reproductive organ adhesion reformation.

It is apparent that more controlled studies need to be performed to adequately evaluate the role of laser, electrocautery, and anti-adhesion adjuvants (Interceed, Gore-Tex®, or Seprafilm) when comparing results with laparoscopy versus laparotomy.

The future of tubal surgery

Tubal factors remain the most common cause of female infertility (approximately one-third of the cases). Surgery, regardless of the technique, for distal tubal disease due to infectious processes results in pregnancy rates of 13–42%. The prognosis for pregnancy following neosalpingostomy is dependent upon:

(1) tubal wall thickness
(2) distal ampullary diameter
(3) health of distal tubal endothelium
(4) extent and type of adhesions

The pregnancy rate varies from 50% to 70% following neosalpingostomy if there are optimal prognostic factors, to 3% for poor prognostic factors. For unfavorable cases, IVF should be initially recommended. Repeat tuboplasties are successful 6–20% of the time.

Successful pregnancies in sheep and rabbits have been reported following tubal transplant with no documented success reported in two human cases, using cyclosporine to avoid tissue rejection in unrelated parties, or in another case of identical twins.

The artificial tube has been used in animals with documented pregnancy success with delivery of normal offspring in rats. However, human use has yet to be successfully tried.

At the present time, improved conception rates appear unlikely with current surgical techniques. A breakthrough with the artificial tube appears to offer limited hope.

Assisted reproductive technology

The majority of women conceive within 12 months of conservative reproductive surgery, except following tubal surgery for post-tubal infectious disease processes. The reported pregnancy rates vary by procedures (Tables 6.1 and 6.2). Assisted reproductive technology (ART) may be considered for the patient with tubal disease primarily for:

(1) inoperable tubal damage
(2) advanced female age
(3) concomitant infertility factors (male, or female endocrine abnormalities)

It has been reported that by life table analysis nearly 70% of women should conceive after four IVF

cycles, which compares favorably with tubal surgery. The Cornell experience demonstrated cumulative pregnancy rates for cycles one to four as: 32%, 59%, 62%, and 75%. However, they published that the per embryo implantation rate declines with age: 29% under age 34, 22% at 34, and 2% at age 44, presumably due to the higher frequency of aneuploidy with advancing age. This finding was also reported by Winston, who in his analysis of 500 patients who had undergone sterilization reversal with at least one tube 6 cm in length found that 15% of women over 40 conceived, versus 75% of younger women. He states that IVF treatment in the United Kingdom is markedly underprovided, and estimates that only 2.5% of the population who would be ideal candidates have been served. Only a handful of those requesting a second cycle in the public sector will get one due to the long waiting lists.

IVF should be complementary to tubal surgery. It is vital to ensure that women who may benefit from IVF do not have effective treatment delayed by ill-advised surgery and that IVF is not the only option offered by physicians who have poor microsurgical or endoscopic technique.

Table 6.1 Pregnancy rates by surgical procedures

Procedure	% Pregnant
Treatment of endometriosis	40–79
Neosalpingostomy	13–42
Fimbrioplasty	60–70
Salpingolysis/ovariolysis	25–62
Tubal reanastomosis	
Sterilization reversal	52–82
Uterotubal junction obstruction	50–69
Repeat tuboplasties	6–20

Table 6.2 Techniques of ART

	IVF	GIFT	ZIFT*
Retrieval Method			
Laparoscopy		X	X
Ultrasound	X		X
Anesthesia			
General		X	X
IV sedation	X		X
Local	X		X
Transfer Method			
Transcervical	X		
Laparoscopy		X	X

*Zygote intrafallopian transfer

What are the ethical implications of shared-risk (refund) programs in ART?

The ethics committee of the American Society for Reproductive Medicine concluded that the shared-risk form for IVF payment may be ethically offered to patients without health insurance. Certain conditions to protect the patients' interests need to be met. These include:

(1) The criterion for success should be clearly defined.
(2) The patients should be fully informed of the financial costs with the advantages and disadvantages fully discussed.
(3) Those patients who do qualify for the program should be fully informed regarding their chance for success, and the program should not guarantee pregnancy and delivery.
(4) The costs of screening and drugs are not to be included.
(5) Those patients who conceive on the first or second cycle should be aware that they are paying a higher cost for IVF than if they had not chosen the shared-risk program.

Proponents of the program, based on the Pacific Fertility Center in San Francisco, California, feel that in specific circumstances physician reimbursement tied to measurable outcomes can be ethically acceptable. Those patients who chose the indemnification program, over traditional payment of fee for service, are able to reduce their financial risk of multiple failures at a fixed cost per failure. Antagonists cite the potential conflicts of interest, which include:

(1) Requiring patients to have additional or repeat testing or adjunctive treatments prior to being approved for the capitation program.
(2) Increasing the likelihood of retrieving more oocytes by using stronger controlled ovarian hyperstimulation.
(3) Transferring more than an optimal number of embryos to help insure success, disregarding the costs and risks of multifetal pregnancies undergoing selective reduction or delivery.

Situations may arise making it difficult to determine whether the clinic should be paid; these include the patient undergoing selective fetal reduction who loses the entire pregnancy in the second trimester and the patient who terminates the pregnancy for chromosomal abnormalities subsequently determined after a 12 week gestation.

Conclusions

(1) Use only a fluid medium with a bare or drawn contact fiber when using the Nd:YAG laser for endometrial ablation or transcervical metroplasty. Use controlled, but rapid movement of the rollerball to reduce the chance of deep thermal injury. Thermachoice uterine balloon therapy may markedly reduce the risk for patients undergoing endometrial ablation to control menorrhagia.

(2) Do not attempt laparoscopic management of ovarian tumors with dense adhesions or if ascites (> 250 cc) is present. Immediately perform a laparotomy or refer to a gynecological oncologist for appropriate treatment of a potential or known malignant tumor.

(3) In conjunction with pelvic exam and ultrasound, Ca-125 is helpful to pre-operatively predict postmenopausal women with ovarian malignancy. Except in women with a familial history of ovarian cancer, its use is questionable for premenopausal women due to other common conditions which may cause false-positive elevation.

(4) Diagnostic laparoscopy with necessary energy sources and instruments available should be scheduled to evaluate the pelvic anatomy in symptomatic patients. Operative laparoscopy may then be performed to treat endoscopically accessible adhesions, endometrial implants, fibroids, and polycystic ovaries. To reduce prolonged operating time and morbidity, patients with extensive disease, especially involving the ureter, bladder, and GI tract, should be rescheduled to undergo microlaser laparotomy. If rectal implants of endometriosis are suspected in patients with an obliterated posterior cul-de-sac, pre-operative evaluation should include a barium enema, sigmoidoscopy, and possibly computed tomography scan. Surgical consultation should be obtained with the surgery scheduled following a bowel preparation.

(5) Laparoscopic assisted vaginal hysterectomy (LAVH) usually offers the patient a more rapid recovery. Since the potential for complications is higher, it is important to appropriately select those patients for this procedure. If operative difficulties are encountered, converting the LAVH to an open laparotomy makes good sense. Each patient should be counseled about this possibility when scheduling the LAVH.

(6) It seems that adhesions reform in spite of our best efforts, whether surgery is performed by laparoscopy or laparotomy and whether lasers or electrocautery are used. Early second-look laparoscopy appears to be the only way to objectively evaluate healing and may be beneficial to reduce the amount of persistent adhesions. Whether this will have a positive effect on conception rates for infertile women, remains to be seen.

(7) Future of tubal surgery. Surgical treatment of distal tubal occlusion is technically easier to perform by microlaser laparotomy for the initial procedure. If repeat tuboplasty is contemplated, as opposed to IVF, the laparoscopic approach is preferred. An endoscopic approach may be used primarily when wishing to relieve the fluid accumulated in hydrosalpinges or when performing salpingectomy for the patient who will be undergoing IVF. When counseling patients regarding the treatment options, consideration should be given to:

1. patient wishes
   a. moral views regarding IVF
   b. anesthesia/surgical approach: ultrasound retrieval, laparoscopy, or laparotomy
2. extent of disease
3. physician skill
   a. tubal surgery (laparoscopy or laparotomy)
   b. IVF conception rates
4. financial resources available, including insurance coverage for:
   a. tubal surgery
   b. IVF
   c. adoption

(8) Assisted reproductive technology. At the present time it still makes sense to attempt to surgically restore normal anatomy, especially in women under age 38. If tubal reocclusion is documented by early second-look laparoscopy or subsequent hysterosalpingogram, IVF should be considered. If the patient has a patent tube and an attempt has been made to correct other fertility factors and conception has not occurred within a year, assisted reproductive technology (ART) should be considered. If male factor infertility cannot be successfully treated by other means, intracytoplasmic sperm injection (ICSI) and IVF with embryo transfer (IVF-ET) should be discussed along with artificial insemination by donor (AID) and adoption.

If the patient is over 35 years old, realistic discussions of the chance for success should be held comparing surgery and ART (Table 6.3). With the advent of the microdose Lupron flare protocol, coupled with assisted hatching, usually IVF-ET is recommended for the patient with diminished ovarian reserve. If the patient has one patent tube and adequate gametes, the author tends to pursue GIFT whenever possible, even following previous tubal surgery after informing the patient that there is a 1% increase incidence in ectopic pregnancy over IVF. Recommendations for ART will vary with each individual center's success rates.

(9) The option for IVF capitation is evolving in an effort to meet a segment of the population's demand for limiting financial risk for multiple failed ART attempts. The ethical issues are complex and remain to be debated. Potential abuses may lead to a lower quality of patient care, decreased credibility for our specialty, and a chance of increased government regulation.

Table 6.3	**ART delivery rates – 40 years and older**	
Age	**IVF**	**GIFT**
40–41	19% (7/37)	38% (6/16)
42–43	27% (3/11)	32% (6/19)
>44	0% (0/7)	11% (1/9)
Total	18% (10/55)	30% (13/44)

Yee, B 1995 and 1996 SART data (used with permission)

Summary

In summary, gynecologists need to delineate how to separate technical feasibility from therapeutic appropriateness, as stated in an 'Obstetrics and Gynecology' editorial by Dr. Roy Pitkin. In other words, just because it can be done, should it be done? Based on the current literature, laparoscopic treatment of ectopic pregnancy, endometriosis, adhesions, and Clomid-resistant polycystic ovaries seems to be justified. When evaluating new techniques, such as laparoscopic assisted vaginal hysterectomy, it is difficult to recommend a change in the standard of care without long-term prospective studies. However, as experience is gained, new standards will emerge. Dr. Pitkin raises the question, 'If we don't critically evaluate our surgical techniques, who will?' As physicians, it is vital to continue to learn and honestly relay this newly gained information to our patients in understandable terms so they may make informed decisions!

BIBLIOGRAPHY

American Society for Reproductive Medicine, Ethics Committee: Shared-risk or refund programs in assisted reproduction. *Fertil Steril* **70**:414–15, 1998.

Andereck W, Thomasma D, Goldworth A, Kushner T: The ethics of guaranteeing patient outcomes. *Fertil Steril* **70**:416–21, 1998.

Baggish MS, Daniell JF: Catastrophic injury secondary to the use of coaxial gas-cooled fibers and artificial sapphire tips for intra-uterine surgery: a report of five cases. *Lasers Surg Med* **9**:581, 1989.

Benadiva C, Kligman I, Davis O, Rosenwaks Z: In vitro fertilization versus tubal surgery: is pelvic reconstructive surgery obsolete? *Fertil Steril* **64**:1051–61, 1995.

Candiani GB, Vercellini P, Fedele L, et al: Conservative surgical treatment for severe endometriosis in infertile women: are we making progress? *Obstet Gynecol Survey* **46**:490–8, 1991.

Challenger RC, Kaufman B: Fatal venous air embolism following sequential unsheathed (bare) and sheathed quartz fiber Nd:YAG laser endometrial ablation. *Anesthesiology* **73**:548, 1990.

Dembo A, Daby M, Stenwig A, et al: Prognostic factors in patients with stage I epithelial ovarian cancer. *Obstet Gynecol* **73**:238, 1990.

Diamond MP, Bradshaw K, Brosens I, Steege J: Current advances in adhesion prevention. Proceedings from the symposium held at the 52nd Annual Meeting of the American Society of Reproductive Medicine, 1996.

Doucette R, Scott J: Comparison of laparoscopically assisted vaginal hysterectomy with abdominal and vaginal hysterectomy. *J Reprod Med* **41**:1–6, 1996.

Eriksson L, Kjellgren O, von Schoultz B: Functional cyst or ovarian cancer: histopathological findings during 1 year of surgery. *Gynecol Obstet Invest* **19**:155–9, 1985.

Gomel V, Taylor P: In vitro fertilization versus reconstructive tubal surgery. *J Assist Reprod Gen* **9**:306–9, 1992.

Hart W, Norris H: Borderline and malignant mucinous tumors of the ovary. *Cancer* **31**:1031, 1973.

Hunter SK, Neeld JB, Scott JR, et al: Developing an artificial fallopian tube: successful in vitral trials in mice. *Fertil Steril* **53**:1083, 1990.

Hur M, Kim J, Moon J, et al: Laparoscopically assisted vaginal hysterectomy. *J Reprod Med* **40**:829–33, 1995.

Jacobs I, Oram D, Fairbanks J, et al: A risk of malignancy index incorporating Ca 125, ultrasound, and menopausal status for the accurate pre-operative diagnosis of ovarian cancer. *Br J Obstet Gynecol* **97**:922, 1991.

Jansen RPS: Early laparoscopy after pelvic operations to prevent adhesions: safety and efficacy. *Fertil Steril* **49**:26, 1988.

Johns A, Diamond M: Laparoscopically assisted vaginal hysterectomy. *J Reprod Med* **39**:424–8, 1994.

Killacky M, Neuwrith R: Evaluation and management of the pelvic mass: a review of 540 cases. *Obstet Gynecol* **71**:319, 1988.

Kirnick S, Kanter MH: Bowel injury from rollerball ablation of the endometrium. *Obstet Gynecol* **79**:833, 1992.

Kliman L, Rome R, Fortune D: Low malignant potential tumors of the ovary: a study of 76 cases. *Obstet Gynecol* **68**:338, 1986.

Maiman M, Seltzer V, Boyce J: Laparoscopic excision of ovarian neoplasms subsequently found to be malignant. *Obstet Gynecol* **77**:563, 1991.

Medical Research International, Society for Assisted Reproductive Technology, The American Fertility Society: In vitro fertilization – embryo transfer (IVF-ET) in the United States: 1990 results from the IVF-ET Registry. *Fertil Steril* **57**:15, 1992.

Morales AJ, Murphy AA: Operative laparoscopy in gynecology. In McLucas B, Morales AJ, Murphy AA (eds): *Current Problems in Obstetrics and Gynecology, and Fertility.* St. Louis, Mosby Year Book, Vol. 15, p 97, 1992.

Munro M, Deprest J: Laparoscopic hysterectomy: does it work?: a bicontinental review of the literature and clinical commentary. *Clin Obstet Gynecol* **38**:401–25, 1995.

Nezhat C, Winer W, Nezhat F: Laparoscopic removal of dermoid cysts. *Obstet Gynecol* **73**:278, 1989.

Nezhat CR, Nezhat FR, Metzger DA, Luciano AA: Adhesion reformation after reproductive surgery by videolaseroscopy. *Fertil Steril* **53**:1008, 1990.

Pitkin RM: Operative laparoscopy: surgical advance or technical gimmick. *Obstet Gynecol* **179**:441, 1992.

Schwartz PE: Ovarian masses: serologic markers. *Clin Obstet Gynecol* **34**:423, 1991.

Scott JR, Hendrickson M, Lash S, et al: Pregnancy after tubo-ovarian transplantation. *Obstet Gynecol* **70**:229, 1987.

Scott R, Silverberg K: Ethics of guaranteeing patient outcomes: a complex issue whose time has not come. *Fertil Steril* **70**:422–4, 1998.

Silverberg KM, Hill GA: Reproductive surgery vs assisted reproductive technology: selecting the correct alternative. *J Gynecol Surg* **7**:67, 1991.

Trimbos-Kemper TCM, Trimbos JB, Vann Hall EV: Adhesion formation after tubal surgery: results of eight-day laparoscopy in 188 patients. *Fertil Steril* **43**:395, 1985.

Tucker SW: Advanced operative laparoscopy in the diagnosis and management of the pelvic mass. In Valle RF, Esposito JM (eds): *Endoscopy in Gynecology – Proceedings of the World Congress of Gynecological Endoscopy, AAGL 18th Annual Meeting.* Santa Springs, American Association of Gynecological Laparoscopists, p 35, 1991.

Tulandi T: Salpingo-ovariolysis: a comparison between laser surgery and electrosurgery. *Fertil Steril* **45**:489, 1986.

Tulandi T, Falcone T, Kafka I: Second-look operative laparoscopy one year following reproductive surgery. *Fertil Steril* **52**:421, 1989.

Winston R: Tubal surgery or in vitro fertilization (IVF)? *J Assist Reprod Gen* **9**:309–11, 1992.

Sources

Key

A CO$_2$ laser
B Nd:YAG laser
C Argon laser
D KTP/532
E Smoke evacuators
F Laser peripherals
G Laparoscopic equipment
H Hysteroscopic equipment
I Insufflators
J Hysteroflators
K Light sources
L Video equipment
M Electrosurgical generators
N Endoscopic sutures, trocars, instruments
O Microscopes
P Adhesion barriers
Q Wallace embryo transfer catheters
R Ovulation induction therapy
S Uterine balloon therapy

Addresses

Bard
8195 Industrial Blvd
Covington, Georgia 30209, USA
Tel. 800 526 4455
N

Cooper Surgical
15 Forest Parkway
Shelton, Connecticut 06484, USA
Tel. 440 946 2453
F,I,J,N,Q

Dexide, Inc.
P.O. Box 980055
Fort Worth, Texas 76118, USA
Tel. 800 645 3378
F

Ethicon, Inc.
P.O. Box 151
Sommerville, New York 08876, USA
Tel. 800 888 9234
N,P

Ferring Pharmaceuticals, Inc.
120 White Plains Road, Suite 400
Tarrytown, New York 10591, USA
Tel. 914 333 8900
R

Genesis, Inc.
1 N. Broadway
Des Plaines, Iowa 60016, USA
Tel. 847 298 3150
G,H,I,J,K,L,M

Genzyme Corporation
5175 South Royal Atlanta Drive
Tucker, Georgia 30084, USA
Tel. 770 496 0952
P

W.L. Gore & Assoc., Inc.
1500 N. 4th St.
Flagstaff, Arizona 86004, USA
Tel. 800 528 8763
P

Gynecare, Inc.
235 Constitution Drive
Menlo Park, California 94015, USA
Tel. 650 614 2500
S

HGM Medical Laser Systems, Inc.
3959 West 1820 South
Salt Lake City, Utah 84104, USA
Tel. 801 972 0500
C

Laserscope
3052 Orchard Drive
San Jose, California 95134, USA
Tel. 800 227 8372
D

Olympus Corp.
2080 Spinger Drive
Lombard, Illinois 60148, USA
Tel. 800 433 1909
G,H,I,J,K,L,M

Organon, Inc.
West Orange
New Jersey 07052, USA
Tel. 973 325 4500
R

Serono Laboratories, Inc.
100 Longwater Circle
Norwell, Massachusetts 02061, USA
Tel. 800 568 4949
R

E.S.C. Sharplan
1 Pearl Court
Allendale, New Jersey 07401, USA
Tel. 201 327 1666
A,B

Sony Corporation of America
Medical Electronics Division
Sony Drive
Park Ridge, New Jersey 07656, USA
Tel. 201 930 7098
L

Karl Storz Co.
600 Corporate Point
Culver City, California 90230, USA
Tel. 800 421 0837
G,H,I,J,K,L,M

Surgimedics
2828 N. Crescent Ridge Drive
The Woodlands, Texas 77381, USA
Tel. 800 669 9001
E

United States Surgical Corp.
141 Glover Ave.
Norwalk, Connecticut 06856, USA
Tel. 800 722 8772
N

Wild Microscopes
Leica Inc.
Surgical Microscope Division
110 Commerce Drive
Allendale, New Jersey 07401, USA
Tel. 800 526 0355
O

WISAP/USA
8305 Melrose Drive
Lenexa, Kansas 66214, USA
Tel. 800 233 8448
G,H,I,J,K,L,M

Richard Wolf Co.
353 Corporate Woods Parkway
Vernon, Illinois 60061, USA
Tel. 800 323 9653
G,H,I,J,K,L,M

Carl Zeiss, Inc.
1 Zeiss Drive
Thornwood, New York 10594, USA
Tel. 914 747 1800
O

Index

Note to reader: Page numbers relating to illustrations (the majority of the entries) are in roman type and indicate the illustration number itself (e.g. 1.4). Page numbers in *italics* are to information in the text (e.g. *155*).